W9-CNL-209

THE
DIABETES
CURE

THE
DIABETES
CURE

THE 5-STEP PLAN TO
ELIMINATE HUNGER,
LOSE WEIGHT,
AND REVERSE DIABETES—
FOR GOOD!

ALEXA FLECKENSTEIN, MD

RODALE

Printed in the United States of America
Rodale Inc. makes every effort to use acid-free ∞, recycled paper ♺.

Throughout the book there are personal testimonials provided by patients. In some cases, the
patients have allowed their actual names to be used, and in others a pseudonym.

Book design by Chris Rhoads

Library of Congress Cataloging-in-Publication Data is on file with the publisher.
ISBN 978–62336–081–8   direct mail hardcover
2   4   6   8   10   9   7   5   3   1   direct mail hardcover

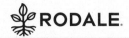

We inspire and enable people to improve their lives and the world around them.
For more of our products, visit **rodalestore.com** or call 800–848–4735.

For my patients,
who taught me more than medical school ever did.

To my husband, Rudolf Jaenisch.

And to my children
Dorothée Berghaus and Johan Jaenisch,
and my granddaughter
Emily Berghaus.

CONTENTS

Part 1

What Is Diabetes?

Part 2

The Impact of Diabetes

Part 3
Curing Your Diabetes

Part 4
Putting It All Together: Plans, Schedules, and Recipes for Your Healthy Life

PREFACE

When did I first recognize the importance of lifestyle to good health? I remember standing over a body in the morgue during my pathology course, and when we searched for the cause of his death, it was simply another case of a heart attack. In medical school we were learning about all of these interesting, rare diseases, but people always seemed to die as a result of what they ate, drank, smoked—basically the way they lived.

That's when it hit me: In all likelihood, my future patients would not die of exotic diseases, but of mundane causes. Sure, the rare diseases were important to know, but it was more important to help my patients live healthier, longer lives. So even before I left medical school, I had developed an interest in treating lifestyles—but no courses were available to satisfy my interest.

During residency, it bothered me that I had to stand by and watch my patients with osteoarthritis clearly deteriorate over time. All I could do was offer painkillers that would corrode their stomachs and damage their livers and kidneys. Medicine seemed to have no interest in determining the cause behind arthritis—doctors and patients alike only aimed to find a pill to make it hurt less. A better pill every year, indeed, but no improvement in the side effect profiles.

Because I had grown up in Europe, where taking herbs, exposing your body to cold water, and eating healthy foods were not "alternative," but mainstream, I took an interest in Natural Medicine. Throughout Europe, physicians recommend these "alternative" methods in their daily practices, and people still use traditional methods today.

During a sabbatical back in Germany, I acquired a degree in Natural Medicine, with the goal of returning to the United States and applying my knowledge back here. As a doctor, I knew that diabetes was related to having high blood sugar. And as a foreigner, I was dismayed by what Americans were eating on a daily basis: cakes with icing, huge bowls of ice cream (our standard size then was about half a cup; here it was half a pint to half a gallon!), doughnuts, cookies five times the size of European cookies, French fries, hamburgers, and all the fast foods that were then much rarer in Europe. And nobody seemed to care for vegetables—*real* food.

As a result, I began treating my patients with the principles of Natural Medicine, and the results were astonishing. Patients were feeling better and leading healthier, happier lives than ever before, and they no longer needed their medications. And this change in health was clearest in my patients who had diabetes. For the longest time it seemed that diabetes was my patients' problem, but it became mine as well when I discovered that I had a gluten intolerance—and gluten is something that instigates inflammation in people affected by it. Suddenly I was a diabetic and grew even more interested in learning about what caused this illness and how to reverse it.

One of the most interesting discoveries of the last 20 years is that chronic inflammation is at the heart of type 2 diabetes,[1] and it dawned on me that traditional Natural Medicine methods had been counteracting those chronic inflammation processes all along! All of the methods I'd been prescribing to my patients had actually been reversing their inflammation and, as a result, fighting—and even curing—their diabetes.

Now I had extra incentive to learn more about the connection between diabetes and inflammation. This book presents many of my findings. As a physician who has treated thousands of patients, I have found that those who chose an anti-inflammatory lifestyle were able to lose weight, come off of their medications, improve their blood sugar, and ultimately cure their diabetes. And I'm glad to say that I'm among them. Now I'd like to share this information with you.

Within this book, you'll discover how inflammation causes type 2 diabetes and how type 2 isn't really a disease at all, but rather a symptom of the inflammation in your body. I'll also provide the tools you need to begin living an anti-inflammatory lifestyle and ultimately cure your diabetes for good (and drop some weight, as well!). Along the way, I'll share some of my patients' success stories, as well as some tips and tricks to help you make the most of your new lifestyle. Because this is a change for life—a life without diabetes!

ACKNOWLEDGMENTS

Thanks to everybody who made me more knowledgeable: Philip Carling, James A. Duke, Dieter Freisenhausen, Harvey Lodish, Sebastian Kneipp (1821–1897), Annemarie Colbin, and so many others who must remain unnamed because of their sheer number. And I am thankful to the members of my writing group for their support: Hung Cheng, Janet McCourt, Anne Mahon, Carol Michael, Gail O'Keefe, Lolita Parker Jr., Jan Preheim, Eleanor Rosellini, Kathryn Silver, Amy Weinberg, and Roanne Weisman.

Without Lora Sickora, my editor at Rodale, this project would not have gotten off the ground: She "found" me and pushed and prodded and nudged me. Thank you, Lora! And my gratitude goes to my agent, Sarah Jane Freymann, for taking me on and believing in this project.

PART 1

What Is Diabetes?

The Real Cause of
Diabetes

∙∙∙

As I see it, every day you do one of two things:
Build health or produce disease in yourself.

—ADELLE DAVIS (1904–1974)

You're in the doctor's office for a routine physical exam when you receive the diagnosis: type 2 diabetes. Sure, you have heard of diabetes before and may even have a general idea of what led to this diagnosis—maybe you have family members with diabetes or have been fighting your weight and a sweet tooth unsuccessfully for years. Or perhaps you've just been living a sedentary lifestyle. In fact, your doctor may have even warned you that in most cases, developing the disease is a direct result of poor nutrition and lack of exercise. But you didn't really listen, because you've been living this way for years and things seemed fine. How did you miss the warning signs? And what exactly went wrong? To find the answer, we need to go back to the basics and look deep inside your body at its building blocks: your cells.

Diabetes and Inflammation

Contrary to popular belief, diabetes is not just the result of having high blood sugar and an insulin-deficient pancreas. Instead, it is a chronic state of widespread inflammation—a direct result of your body not being used to its original

3

design. We have ancient bodies and ancient souls, and in these modern times, we don't use them in the way in which they were intended. The little-acknowledged truth is that our bodies are made for outdoor living (i.e., hunting and gathering), not for sitting in a cubicle day in and day out, eating fabricated "food," and watching TV until late in the night. Did you ever think that this kind of lifestyle hurts your body—and that it deprives you of productivity, creativity, and happiness?

Risk Factors for Type 2 Diabetes

There are several risk factors linked to the development of diabetes. Take a look at the list below to determine how many apply to you.

- **Family history.** Both your genes and your childhood environment (learned eating habits, outdoor activities, sleeping patterns, reward mechanisms, etc.) can increase or decrease your risk of developing diabetes.

- **Weight and fat distribution.** The more fat you have (especially around your middle), the more resistant your body becomes to insulin and the hunger-regulating hormone leptin.

- **Sedentary lifestyle.** Prolonged periods of sitting increase your chances of developing diabetes. Why? Working your muscles squelches the fire of inflammation. Not using your muscles leads to the development of diabetes. And when you sit, you barely use any muscles.

- **Race.** Certain races are more prone to the ravishments of the Western diet than others: Hispanics, blacks, Hawaiians, Native Americans, and Asians have an increased risk of developing diabetes.

- **Age.** Beginning at age 45, your risk for diabetes grows considerably. At this time in your life, you have likely eaten too many cupcakes with icing and walked too few miles—and the effects of this lifestyle are beginning to show. And retirees have an even higher risk of developing diabetes because they can easily fall prey to the damages of a sedentary lifestyle.

- **Gestational diabetes.** Diabetes during pregnancy is like an early warning shot: You have the genes, and if you are not careful with what you eat and how you live, you will eventually develop diabetes.

You may wonder how so many different things go haywire in a diabetic's body, all seemingly unconnected, like high blood pressure, arthritis, and cancer. What is the unifying process underlying all of those divergent diseases? It is *inflammation*. And a January 2013 meta-analysis of 10 studies with more than 19,000 participants showed that raised levels of inflammation markers were significantly associated with an increased risk of having type 2 diabetes.[1]

- **Giving birth to a large baby.** Having a baby who weighs more than 9 pounds puts you at risk for developing diabetes later in life.

- **Prediabetes.** When your hemoglobin A1c hovers close to 6.0, consider yourself at risk.

- **An overweight peer group.** People have a tendency to adopt the lifestyle habits of those closest to them, including family members, friends, and co-workers.

- **Hypothyroidism.** An elevated TSH (thyroid-stimulating hormone) level and/or antibodies against thyroid tissue are often found in patients with diabetes. And many have gluten intolerance. Be sure your doctor addresses all of these problems.

- **High blood pressure.** This is part of the metabolic syndrome (overweight, hypertension, high lipids, and insulin resistance), so having one of them sets you up for developing the rest.

- **Polycystic Ovary Syndrome (PCOS).** This syndrome manifests itself more in your ovaries and your skin, but it still has many features of diabetes. And the treatment is also the same: improved lifestyle.

- **A history of stroke.** If you've experienced a stroke, your odds of developing diabetes automatically increase.

- **Acanthosis nigricans.** This is a skin condition in which skin located under the armpits and in folds of the body is dark, thicker, and velvety.

- **Gluten intolerance.** Those who are gluten intolerant are at an increased risk of developing diabetes as well.

- **Poor sleeping habits.** Lack of sleep promotes weight gain and obesity.

Included in this meta-analysis was a 2001 study published in the *Journal of the American Medical Association* showing that the levels of interleukin-6 and C-reactive protein (two of the major markers of inflammation) were considerably higher in women who subsequently developed diabetes.[2] Researchers found that women with higher baseline levels of interleukin-6 were at 7.5 times greater risk of becoming diabetic than those with the lowest levels of inflammation. Furthermore, women with higher levels of C-reactive protein were at 15.7 times greater risk of developing diabetes. After adjusting their findings for known risk factors, the researchers reported that the women with the highest levels of interleukin-6 were 2.3 times more likely to become diabetics, while those with highest levels of C-reactive protein were 4.2 times more likely to develop diabetes.

But where does all of the inflammation come from? This widespread and sneaky inflammation stems from an accumulation of fat and waste debris in and around every cell in your body that affects every single organ in your body. It also prevents your mitochondria (those specialized subunits in all of your cells that produce energy like little batteries) from generating the energy you need. Mitochondria are intimately involved in the insulin secretion process and are affected negatively by a too-nutritious (or high-calorie) diet. As a result, your damaged mitochondria hinder proper insulin secretion, which leads to the development of diabetes.[3] And sooner or later, the breakdown of your mitochondria will cause all kinds of other diseases as well, including heart disease, stroke, and even cancer.

How you choose to live your life either increases or decreases the inflammation in your body. Every day—every moment—you are making a decision to either put out the fire of inflammation or stoke it.

Inflammation: Acute versus Chronic

Have you ever had an area on your body that's painful, red, swollen, and hot? These are the classic four cardinal signs of inflammation, established by the Roman physician Celsus (circa 25 BC to 50). And in the second century AD, Galen (129 AD to circa 200 AD) added a fifth: penuria, which means loss of function.

In an acute infection, such as a bee sting, an infected tooth, or an acutely inflamed knee, all five signs are often there. In chronic inflammation, those signs may be harder to spot, mainly because the inflammatory process takes

What Role Does Genetics Play?

Many people blame their diabetes on their genes: "I just have bad genes. After all, my mother and my grandmother had diabetes, too."

On one level they are right: You can weigh 300 pounds and as long as you don't have a genetic predisposition, you will never develop diabetes. Genes and their DNA carry the blueprint for everything that we have inherited and everything that makes up our bodies. Certain genes can increase your risk of developing diabetes, while other genes can cause you to gain weight more easily than other people.

Your genome—the strand of DNA in each cell that carries all your genes and some junk DNA, the non-gene "empty" areas between genes—is so well packed that in each cell, only the parts that are urgently needed are exposed to the surface. The rest is tucked away. (In a liver cell, for example, everything that pertains to your heart or your hair color is stowed away and only the liver genes are exposed.)

What we are learning is that, on one level, the junk DNA and the packaging is even more important than the original strand of DNA. And this packaging (called epigenetics) is influenced by lifestyle factors, such as what you eat (and even what your mother ate), how often you exercise, and how much you sleep.[4] So, in a way, you are responsible for your own genes because you can influence them—to a certain degree. Further, some scientists think that your lifestyle influences most of your total health outcome, including your epigenetic packaging, *especially* if your mother and your grandmother had diabetes![5] So while you may not be able to change your genes, you can change your lifestyle and, subsequently, your epigenetics. And you can even hand these epigenetic changes down to your children and grandchildren.

place inside your body and is, therefore, less visible. But even though you can't see it, this chronic inflammation is causing insidious damage inside your body.

Once you are told that having chronic inflammation in your body leads to the development of numerous health problems such as diabetes, you may

(continued on page 10)

Triggers of Inflammation

Below is a list of the wide range of triggers that can incite the white blood cell response and the cascade of chemical processes of inflammation.

- Alcohol
- Allergens
- Artificial colors and flavors
- Bacteria
- Burns
- Chemicals
- Dairy
- Dirt
- Drugs
- Exercise: Both too much and too little can be harmful.
- Fats: Certain dietary fats heal, while others cause harm.
- Frostbite
- Fungi
- Herbicides
- Insulin: Although we need insulin to process dietary sugars, too much insulin damages your cells.
- Molds
- Molecules: Certain molecules are foreign to your body, such as some modern drugs and food additives.
- Obesity
- Parasites
- Pesticides
- Pollutants

- Preservatives: Man-made preservatives are often damaging, whereas plant-derived preservatives like curry, which is used in India to preserve food, are beneficial in lower doses. Often, they are antioxidants.

- Radiation

- Rancid foods

- Skin irritants

- Sleep: Not getting enough sleep is harmful to our bodies on many levels.

- Stress: There is good stress and bad stress. Take the example of antioxidants, which are not just superbly beneficial compounds. Plants manufacture antioxidants when germs and insects nibble on their leaves. These antioxidants act as weapons against invaders and kill unwanted pests. When we consume small amounts of antioxidants in our food, our bodies send small stress signals to fight off the compounds. These stress signals stimulate our immune systems and cause them to function at a better rate. But in larger doses, antioxidants can cause us harm as well. So good stress comes from things like cold showers, limited exposure to antioxidants, and small amounts of exercise, while bad stress results from too little sleep, too much exercise (or none at all), unlimited exposure to antioxidants, and bland, processed foods.

- Sugars, especially HFCS (high-fructose corn syrup)

- Sunlight: Finding the right balance of exposure to natural sunlight is important—both getting too much and getting too little can be harmful.

- Toxins

- Trauma

- Viruses

- Wounds

naturally want to expel all inflammation from your body. After all, if it causes diabetes, it is as desirable as a case of head lice or bedbugs. But as hot and raging as inflammation is, it is also an extremely useful tool in your body. Without it, nothing could heal in your body—not even a simple scratch. You're already aware of the inflammation that occurs from infection (when white blood cells and cascades of chemical processes rid your body of intruders such as viruses, bacteria, and fungi). But infection is only one example of inflammation.

Inflammation protects you from germs, foreign bodies, and a host of other dangers, and it is the reason that a cut will heal in a timely manner. But imagine if this hot and raging swelling takes place in your joints, your heart, your brain, your kidneys, and your liver. It's invisible to you because this kind of inflammation only occurs deep inside your body where it can't be seen. You can feel it, though, in all those aches, pains, and discomforts you experience. They are signals that something is wrong and inflamed, even if your doctor can't find a fitting diagnosis. And this ongoing, chronic inflammation is the kind that you don't want to have smoldering in your body.

How Inflammation Works

To explain how inflammation works, let's look at an example of acute inflammation. When a splinter lodges in your finger, your body immediately begins to build a wall of inflammation around it by attracting white blood cells to the site of the splinter. The white blood cells gobble up the germs and toxins that otherwise would spread throughout your entire body. Once the white blood cells are filled with toxins, they die. And this mass of dead cells is called pus. Next, your skin breaks and the splinter is expelled from your finger, along with the pus. Then the tissue closes and your skin heals over.

Sounds straightforward, right? Well, it's actually a bit more complicated than that. For inflammation to work, an intricate dance between blood cells and plasma proteins (also known as mediator chemicals) has to ensue. If germs invade your body and your body cannot mount an inflammatory defense, you will die.

An intruding germ carries chemicals on its surface that the body recognizes as foreign. And defense starts immediately: These invaders attract the two prongs of inflammation—cells and biochemicals—that trigger the intricate cascade of recognizing the invader, mounting the forces, attacking, ingesting, destroying, and cleaning up. Then the healing begins.

First, the blood vessels around the pathogens dilate to bring more blood to the site, and arriving with the blood are white blood cells (the defenders) and mediator chemicals (the messengers). The enlarged vessels seep plasma (the watery part of blood) into the surrounding areas until only the white blood cells are left, packed tightly in the capillaries. Now you have a swollen wall around the germs. The mediator chemicals have numerous supportive functions such as attracting more white blood cells, dilating the vessels even more, producing heat so that germs are killed, and stimulating the nerve endings susceptible to pain. Feeling pain is important for two reasons: to call attention to the fact that something is wrong and to remind you to keep the affected body part still. If you didn't feel pain, you would go on with your busy life and your body would have a harder time healing.

After the germs are killed and devoured, and that painful splinter has been expelled, this complicated cascade of mediator chemicals and blood cells has run its course, and the chemicals terminate the process until everything is quiet and healthy again. There is an end to the inflammatory process. But with diabetes, there is no end. The inflammation goes on and on because the triggers can't be ejected as easily as that one splinter. Instead, triggers are everywhere. Take a look at "Triggers of Inflammation" on page 8. What do these triggers have in common? They are all either old enemies of ours, like germs and invading bacteria, or they are "unnatural" new chemicals—if we define natural by how we lived through millions of years of evolution before modern life started to upset our balances.

Inflammation is a fire in your body that cleanses the premises. It is a useful, gentle, controlled incineration—until it becomes a chronic smoldering fire that destroys your body cell by cell. Modern chemistry has invented molecules that humans have never before encountered in all of evolution, and those modern molecules are affecting our health. If you look at the offending list, you may wonder how it's possible to avoid all of these things that are in the very air we breathe, pollute our waters, and contaminate our soils. And you are right: We cannot avoid all triggers of inflammation. But that doesn't mean we are helpless. We can start with a few things that are within our control! Diabetes can be reversed by quenching the inflammation in your body and restarting your sluggish metabolism.

Interestingly, most of the inflammation in your body begins in your intestines.[6] Your bowels are where the world and you meet intimately: You take up foodstuff—the future building blocks of your cells—right there where gut wall and blood connect. And even more interestingly, the gut-related immune system comprises about 70 percent or more of your entire immune system, which means you can't overestimate the importance of unknown processes in your bowels. There, chronic inflammation begins, and from there you are able to heal.

Is Diabetes Really a
Disease?

∙∙∙

It is no measure of health
to be well adjusted
to a profoundly sick society.

—JIDDU KRISHNAMURTI (1895–1985)

There is no doubt about it: Type 1 diabetes (also called juvenile diabetes) is a disease. It strikes unexpectedly and stems from a single defect over which we have no control—insulin deficiency. And insulin, the hormone that regulates the amount of sugar circulating in your bloodstream, is vitally important because too much sugar in concentrated form is highly damaging to your cells. During the development of type 1 diabetes, specific insulin-producing pancreatic cells (known as beta cells) die as a result of genetic, viral, and/or autoimmune disorders. And nothing can make those dead beta cells function again. The dying or dead cells stop producing insulin, leaving the body without an insulin supply. This increases blood sugar levels and ultimately poisons all of your body's cells. Without the use of biosynthetic (or man-made) insulin, this poisoning would result in death.

Type 2 diabetes (also called adult-onset diabetes) is a very different story because even though you may have a genetic predisposition, you also have

13

an opportunity to rehabilitate your abysmal metabolism by changing the lifestyle that brought you to this diagnosis in the first place! If a doctor would say, "Your lifestyle is sick" every time he diagnosed someone with type 2 diabetes, we would soon overcome this deathly epidemic. But most physicians are not trained to do this. And those who are want to spare their patients' feelings.

Initially, before your official diagnosis of type 2 diabetes, you don't lack insulin. But eventually your poor dietary and lifestyle choices will lead to chronic inflammation inside your body and will raise your blood sugar. This inflammation begins as a coping mechanism for your cells: They're trying to heal themselves. Inflammation is the by-product of cells ridding themselves of toxins and germs. But the inflammation soon becomes overwhelming for your cells, and your pancreas begins to produce more and more insulin in an attempt to lower your blood sugar. This has two consequences: First, your pancreatic cells become exhausted, unable to meet your body's high demand for insulin. And second, your body's cells just don't respond to insulin properly because high levels of insulin have been floating around and "knocking at the door" of your cells too often. As a result, your cells become *insulin resistant*, which means they require higher and higher levels of insulin in order to respond.

Because high blood sugar levels are toxic and dangerous, your pancreatic beta cells crank out more and more insulin—until they are utterly spent. When this happens, type 2 diabetics have to take insulin because their own production does not meet the demand anymore. Giving insulin to people who have insulin resistance and, therefore, need more than the natural amount their bodies can provide, has two results:

1. Insulin functions like a growth factor—and lets cancer cells grow.[1]
2. Insulin locks fat in those people's cells, which basically makes them gain weight or, at a minimum, hinders weight loss.[2]

Why does this happen? Insulin was intended for use in people with type 1 diabetes and was never meant for those who are overfed and underexercised. You may find that taking certain medications could improve your condition to a degree, but once you begin taking insulin, the situation has already gone too far, and it is time to rein it in.

Type 2 Diabetes Is *Not* a Disease

If your type 2 diabetes isn't a disease like type 1, what is it? Type 2 diabetes is a state of insulin waste—a direct result of the havoc the wrong lifestyle wreaks on your body. Long before any doctor calls it a "disease," your blood sugar is on the rise and inflammation is smoldering inside your body. And as multiple studies have shown, this inflammation begins affecting your brain, skin, gums, teeth, lungs, heart, bones, stomach, esophagus, liver, kidneys, gut, pancreas, breasts, ovaries, testicles, penis, vagina, eyes, ears, taste, sinuses, muscles, joints and tendons, arteries, veins, peripheral nerves, and lymphatic system.[3-32]

The development of type 2 diabetes begins when you eat something sugary for the first time in your life.[33] You may not become sick right away, but at that moment, something changes inside your body—and not for the better. The inflammation begins and your taste buds (and your gut) suddenly have different expectations: They crave something sweet, and they expect to receive something sweet again. Or the development of type 2 diabetes can start when you marry your sweetheart, have two kids, and find that you are so tired in the evening that all you can do is sit in front of the TV. No, you are not sick the very next day, but again, something in your body has changed.[34] You begin to slump while seated, and soon you notice the development of belly fat.

Type 2 is the *preventable* kind of diabetes—or the kind that comes with "civilization" and with overeating. (In times of famine, very few cases occur.) But although it is preventable, and even curable, the truth is that physicians diagnose diabetes too late because they focus on the point where the diabetes test turns positive, not on the subtle changes that happen in the patient before he becomes overtly ill. This is probably a big part of the reason why many diabetics already have end-organ disease at the time of diagnosis.

The Role of Insulin in Type 2 Diabetes

Doctors are offering insulin against these self-inflicted ills, too, as if type 2 diabetes were like type 1. But, as we said, insulin was never meant to cure an overfed, underexercised body, and it is a short-term solution—if any at all.

Not moving enough and eating sugary, starchy junk food fills your cells with fat and debris. Insulin, in order to work, needs to latch on to receptors on the cell walls. The receptors then signal to the cell what to do with the accumulated sugar. If you fill your cells with fat and debris, they cannot respond as well to the signals insulin sends them.

How to Measure Diabetes

There are five main tests used to diagnose type 2 diabetes.

1. **Spot blood sugar.** Since blood sugar can quickly rise and fall, depending on what and when you ate, this is a very unreliable test. But if you don't have any suspicious symptoms, this test may be all you need. Of course, if you have already been diagnosed with diabetes, your doctor can do more reliable tests in the offlce.

   On the other hand, if you have prediabetes, it is a good idea to have a meter at home to help monitor your blood sugar levels. Don't get nervous about every small aberration in your sugar levels. Look at the big picture: Are the numbers going in the right direction, or are they all over the map? This will help you to determine your dietary needs and how frequently you should meet with your physician.

2. **Fasting blood sugar.** While this test is cheap, fast, and requires only a small bit of blood, the results can vary depending on what you ate the day before. However, if your fasting numbers are consistently high, you should pay attention!

3. **Oral glucose tolerance test.** A complicated procedure where the patient drinks an incredibly sweet fluid before having blood drawn at half-hour intervals, this test is designed to ascertain how fast the sugar load is cleared out of your bloodstream. While it's complicated and time-consuming for the patient, it was probably the most accurate test until the A1c came along.

4. **A1c (also known as hemoglobin A1c or glycated hemoglobin).** Every time you eat sugar, your body adds

Once you understand what is happening in your body when type 2 diabetes strikes, you'll also understand that taking pills and insulin will never eliminate the root cause. Really, there is no other way to heal than by ridding your body of the inflammation that caused your diabetes.

sugar molecules to a hemoglobin protein in your red blood cells. This buildup of molecules lasts the entire life span of the red blood cell, which is roughly 3 months. A1c is an easy blood test that measures how much sugar you ate over the previous few months. Conventionally, if a patient's A1c returns at 6.4 or higher, he or she is diagnosed with diabetes, while an A1c of 5.7 to 6.3 shows that the patient has prediabetes.[35]

I believe the A1c is the best diabetes test because it ignores the ebb and flow of sugars throughout the day as we eat. While the rise and fall of blood sugar is visible in the test, these changes present as a gradual increase or decrease instead of jumping all over the place. It also has an added benefit: You don't need to fast for an A1c test.

5. **Insulin and insulin resistance.** If you show signs of abdominal fat and have high spot blood sugar, but your insulin level is normal or low, it means that your pancreas is becoming exhausted and your insulin resistance should be measured via a blood test. If your insulin levels are too high, your pancreas is churning out insulin as fast as it can to fight those dangerous blood sugar spikes. No further testing needed at this point, because your doctor will automatically know you are in trouble.

If you have insulin resistance, your body requires higher and higher levels of insulin to lower your blood sugar. At this stage, you are in grave danger of burning out your pancreas altogether and needing insulin shots for the rest of your life.

Diabetes and Metabolic Syndrome

Conventional physicians define diabetes as impaired glucose control. But impaired glucose control is only one of the many facets of diabetes. Disturbed fat metabolism (abnormal lipids), decreased microcirculation, poor mitochondrial function, and decreased immune function are also factors.[36-39] Simply put, there is more to diabetes than meets the eye: It is a systemic problem that involves the whole body. And conventional medicine has begun to acknowledge this with the diagnosis of metabolic syndrome, also known as syndrome X.

Metabolic syndrome as a term concedes that type 2 diabetes does not come alone, but travels with a host of difficulties. By calling it a syndrome instead of a disease, conventional physicians are approaching the treatment of diabetes in a more holistic way, showing that it is not a "disease" like any other.

Metabolic syndrome and syndrome X are still only names and definitions. They don't convey what's really going on inside your body—the enormous fatigue, the constant cravings, the cellulite, and the organ shutdowns that happen one after the other because they have not been used.

About half of the US population has at least one of the conditions that compose metabolic syndrome:

- Diabetes (high blood sugar)
- Hypertension (high blood pressure)
- Hyperlipidemia (high blood fats)
- Central obesity (a big belly)

Recently, research pointed to another condition as well:

- Uricemia (high uric acid)

So how is uric acid related to type 2 diabetes? High dietary fructose elevates uric acid, and this blocks the availability of nitric oxide (a free radical).[40] Insulin needs nitric oxide to reduce blood sugar, so it makes sense that high uric acid from high fructose hinders insulin from doing its proper work, which ultimately increases your risk of developing diabetes. (A word of caution: Free radicals are involved in essential life functions. But freely roaming free radicals—those not quenched immediately—make for early aging and inflammation in your body. As in so many biological mechanisms, free radicals need to be finely balanced—not too much, not too little. If they aren't broken

David's Story

David came to me because his primary care physician had urged him to start high blood pressure pills, and he was reluctant. He had heard that those medications were notorious for causing impotence, which scared him. A successful stockbroker, David divulged that his work was his life. He admitted to having a sedentary lifestyle, grabbing food on the go, and attending many dinner functions that involved heavy alcohol consumption.

It was easy to see how his life was out of balance: too much food, some really bad nutritional choices—like his habit of eating salty potato chips in the car—no exercise, not enough sleep, an endless workload, and so on. His blood pressure was 170/95, and his labs showed his total cholesterol elevated at 260, with his "good" cholesterol measuring too low and his triglycerides too high. But that wasn't all. When David's test results came back, he was surprised to hear my diagnosis: type 2 diabetes. (Other physicians may have diagnosed this as syndrome X.)

I promptly explained that his condition was reversible—if he chose to change his habits and rid his body of the inflammation that caused his problems. And once he understood how his lifestyle was related to his diagnosis, David became proactive: He hired a personal trainer to guide him through using the machines in his company's workout room, which he had never used before. He also talked his wife into serving more anti-inflammatory foods at home, which renewed their relationship: Discovering new healthy foods became their first common project in a long time. At business dinners, he chose smaller portions and substituted fish and filling vegetables in place of fried foods and dairy.

Soon, David found himself bringing home less work. Instead, he would spend his free time by going on a short walk with his wife after dinner each night. Within the year, David lost 30 pounds, which only encouraged him to continue with his new lifestyle and push himself a little more. Soon after, David's blood pressure normalized and, best of all, he had reversed his diabetes. With his newfound energy, David finally had a routine that he could maintain and a new relationship to enjoy with his wife.

down fast, free radicals invade your cells, target your DNA, and damage it, seemingly on a quest to destroy what comes into their path. Eating the wrong foods, pollution of all kinds (including some of the medications your doctor prescribes you), ingesting nonfoods such as heavy metals—these all add to the free radical burden. This burden grows as we age. But an anti-inflammatory diet can help to reduce the burden.

Diabetes and Weight

Feel your belly right now. If it is bulging, you are overweight. (On some level you probably knew it all along.) You can stand on a scale or calculate your body mass index (BMI) online at www.exrx.net/calculates/BMI.html to get an idea of whether or not your weight is contributing to your diabetes, but neither of these methods will provide the whole picture. The scale doesn't account for your height, while the BMI calculation presumes an average amount of muscle and fat. As a result, it can overestimate adiposity (fattiness) in a healthy athlete with thick muscles and underestimate the obesity of an older person with little muscle mass.

While it's good to check your weight every morning and know your BMI (the normal range is 18.5 to 24.9), neither one can detect the riskiest fat in your body: belly fat. If you have a protruding stomach at all (and it's not due to water or gas, which might signal food intolerances), you are at a higher risk

Waist-to-Hip Ratio

Measure your waist at the height of your belly button. Next, measure around your hips. If your BMI is a bit on the high side and your waist is quite a bit smaller than your hips, you probably have more muscle than fat. This means you are not in danger of developing diabetes. But if your abdomen is bigger than (or nearly as big as) your hips, you'd better pay attention.

To find your waist-to-hip ratio, divide your waist measurment by your hip measurment. A healthy waist-to-hip ratio should be lower than 0.95 in men and 0.80 in women. A ratio of 1:1 in men and 0.85:1 in women is where trouble begins, putting you at high risk for diabetes and heart disease.

for developing diabetes. Therefore, measuring your waist circumference is really the best test. And grabbing your belly is the easiest way to determine whether your waist circumference is of concern.

Physicians used to think that a slab of belly fat was like lard in the pantry: unmovable, unchanged, forever. Now they have found that belly fat is extremely active, like a stealth factory churning out secret molecules that make people eat more and build up more fat.[41] This is why abdominal fat kills: You become compact by taking in more calories than you're spending.

While I don't want you to count calories, you need to know that fat comes from food. There is no secret fat manufacturer in your body that somehow surreptitiously manufactures fat. And there are certainly no evil genes. Your genes do not determine how you build up fat, but instead why you eat so much. With certain genes, you are simply drawn to eat more and move less.

Weight Loss Is Necessary

The answer to curing diabetes does not lie in a miracle pill or a miracle diet. The only way you can cure your diabetes is by changing your lifestyle and losing that belly fat one step at a time, because belly fat is an inflammation hot spot. I won't promise that you will lose 200 pounds within a year by following my plan because science has proven that fast weight loss very rarely lasts.[42] And no, you will never be able to go back to your old ways—but why would you want to? This is not a temporary fad; it is a permanent change. And you will love it! By taking it one step at a time, you will reverse your diabetes, lose weight, and keep it off for the rest of your life.

The best news? You can start today, because the longer you procrastinate, the harder it will be to take control of your health and your weight. Every pound you gain, you'll have to shed later. And here's another reason why you shouldn't postpone your weight loss: A recent study shows that your fitness in midlife predicts how healthy you'll be and what diseases you'll have in old age.[43] Here are three facts.

- **Diabetes can kill you.** It leads to heart attacks, strokes, blindness, impotence (and sexual dysfunction in women), amputations, cancer, arthritis, depression, mood swings, kidney failure, and many more unpleasant conditions.
- **Type 2 diabetes is curable if you work on it.** At least in its earlier stages. And in its later stages, you can stave off the horrible decline with a better lifestyle.

- **Hard work has a bad reputation.** We think everything should come easy: the ready-to-eat TV dinner, the shirt that doesn't need ironing, the car that carries us everywhere. In reality, hard work gives us satisfaction, which is, in the long run, more important and rewarding than the easy "happiness" we get out of an "easy" lifestyle.

But here is what is possible.

- If you are prediabetic, you can avoid getting overt diabetes.
- If you have mild to moderate diabetes, you can reduce the burden of disease and even be cured.
- If you are already on insulin, you will likely not be cured, but you may be able to reduce your insulin units or even stop taking insulin altogether. (Be sure to consult with your doctor first!)

Have you done everything you can to turn your diabetes around? Or have you been a nice patient, taken your pills like the doctor told you, and done nothing otherwise? In conventional drug studies, diabetes often is called "controlled" if the person's blood sugar stays within the limits of 7.0 to 10.0 A1c. We can be sure that at those numbers, the damage done by high blood sugar is continuing in the body. I personally favor an approach that does not "manage" the patient's diabetes, but gets rid of it. And in many cases it can be done, with a well-rounded, natural approach—and determination on the patient's side.

Sure, there may be obstacles in your way. But I'm going to show you how to slowly but surely overcome those obstacles. At no point will I tell you that it is easy. But I promise that it is doable if you know how. My patients have done it, and they've proven that it works.

Thin and Diabetic

Research has shown that overweight diabetics live longer than thin diabetics.[44] Based on this, researchers concluded that "somehow" fat might be protective, after all. But don't be fooled into thinking your fat is protecting you. The study did not take gluten intolerance into account.

Our modern degenerative diseases have to do with four main culprits: wheat, dairy, sugar, and trans fats. Traditionally, about 10 percent of people with type 2 diabetes have been slim,[45] and their underlying condition could be gluten intolerance, a disease where the bowels are chronically inflamed because common foods like wheat, barley, rye, and oats are toxic to them, which leads to a lower body weight. Sprue, celiac sprue, celiac disease, and gluten intolerance are all different names for the same disease—the one that turns your daily bread into poison.

About 1 in 10 people cannot digest gluten well. If you have red or blonde hair, blue eyes, and/or fair skin, you have a higher chance of being gluten intolerant,[46] though I have certainly seen the disease in dark-haired people as well. There is no cure for celiac disease. The only recourse is to eliminate all gluten from your diet. Some people have a hard time letting go of breads, cookies, cakes, and pastas. But once you realize that you can eat brown rice, beans, lentils, and chickpeas as much as you want, you'll suddenly find that you are not only disease free, but also living a healthier life, because much of our junk food is based on wheat (combined with fat, salt, and sugar).

Sometimes late-onset type 1 diabetes can be misdiagnosed as type 2. Those misdiagnosed type 1 patients and undiagnosed cases of gluten intolerance might account for the rising number of slim diabetics. Gluten intolerance, type 1 diabetes, and type 2 diabetes seem to be increasing—a likely result of the adulterated foods we eat, our sick environment, and newer hybrids of wheat that have a higher gluten content per kernel.[47]

People with no immune tolerance for gluten might get diarrhea, skin rashes, bloating, and suffer all kinds of neurologic and psychiatric symptoms. Half of the symptoms are not showing in their bellies, which is one reason gluten intolerance is still one of the most widely underdiagnosed diseases, even though awareness has increased within the last 10 years. So, if you have been diagnosed with type 2 diabetes recently and are not overweight, talk to your doctor to see if you could be a misdiagnosed type 1 diabetic or if you could have a gluten problem.

In short, being thin while being a diabetic is not good news: You might be thin because your intestines are not able to take essential nutrients from the foods you eat, which means your body is deprived like that of a starving person. Gluten intolerance creates a state of constant inflammation in your bowels, and very likely in many other organs, as well. When you think about it, it's no wonder that gluten intolerance can cause diabetes with its constant gut inflamation.

PART 2

The Impact of Diabetes

Diabetes
and Its Unpleasant Consequences

From the bitterness of disease
man learns the sweetness of health.

—CATALAN PROVERB

Worldwide, an estimated 371 million people are afflicted with the metabolic derangement we call type 2 diabetes—a number greater than the entire population of the United States—and nearly half of them are unaware of their condition.[1] In the United States, roughly 10 percent of Americans have diabetes, a third of whom remain undiagnosed.[2] And between the prescribed medications, strokes, heart attacks, amputations, dialysis, and other complications, type 2 diabetes is the most expensive health care issue in the country.[3] It has become an epidemic—and almost anyone can be stricken. Think about it: You probably know at least a few people who have been diagnosed with diabetes.

The elderly constitute the largest group: More than 25 percent of our senior population has type 2 diabetes.[4] But while it's easy to think of diabetes as an old-age affliction, that's simply no longer the case. Sadly, obesity is now being diagnosed in young children (including toddlers),[5] and diabetics are now dying younger than ever before—succumbing to poor health during the years that should be the most productive of their lives—while those who are fortunate enough to make it through their younger years face a life filled with diabetic complications, and possibly even medication.

The Pros and Cons of Diabetes Medications

It is so easy for a doctor to take out her prescription pad—and so much easier for a patient to take some pills for the rest of her life than face the hard task of turning her life around and making it healthier. We are a culture of pill poppers; we want problems to go away, and fast. After all, we have more important things to do than work on a lifestyle of health and happiness. And because of that, we are sick.

Do you experience nausea, anxiety, seizures, depression, or loss of appetite? And have you ever wondered if these occurrences are caused by your diabetes medication? Every single pill you take has side effects, and this includes your diabetes pills. This does not mean that you should stop taking your medication. (Always consult with your doctor.) But when your doctor suggests a new pill, think of it as an offer (not an order), and ask questions. Make yourself knowledgeable by asking your doctor or your pharmacist about the pros and cons of each medication you're prescribed so you'll know exactly what to expect from it.

Anti-Diabetic Drugs

Medications prescribed to fight diabetes come from different drug families, lower blood sugar through different mechanisms, and are often given together. These drug families are listed below to give you an idea of the benefits and side effects you can expect while taking each type.

Biguanides lower blood sugar by increasing insulin sensitivity. The most commonly prescribed biguanide, a generic medication called metformin, lowers blood sugar in two ways: It prevents new sugar production in your liver and removes sugar from your bloodstream by shifting it into your muscles, rendering the sugar harmless. (The medical community still isn't sure how metformin does it, as the exact mechanism is not yet understood.) In turn, the lowered blood sugar returns insulin sensitivity to your cells. Metformin is, therefore, an insulin-sparing drug. By lowering sugars in the blood, metformin also squelches inflammation, as sugars are inflammatory. This medication also hinders cancer formation and cancer growth by interrupting the sugar production in your liver: Without glucose for fuel, cancer cells can't thrive.

Because of its blood sugar–lowering effect, metformin also seems to have anti-inflammatory action in several organs and diseases, and it has been used to treat polycystic ovary syndrome (PCOS), metabolic syndrome, and cancer.[6-8] This sounds impressive, but a 2012 placebo-controlled study published in the *European Journal of Endocrinology* compared the effectiveness of metformin against berberine (a chemical derived from plants such as barberry, goldenseal, and goldenthread) in the treatment of PCOS and found that berberine not only outperformed metformin in the treatment of PCOS, but also benefited the subjects' waist lines.[9] Researchers found that the waist circumference of women treated with berberine decreased almost twice as much as those treated with metformin. Also, the waist-to-hip ratio in the berberine group decreased 7 percent, a significantly greater reduction than the 3 percent reduction observed in the metformin group. And while metformin rarely causes hypoglycemia or weight gain, a meta-analysis of 13 trials did not show much in the line of reduced mortality or cardiovascular morbidity.[10] For a drug so widely used, this is a poor result.

In rare cases, this medication can cause lactic acidosis in people with diabetes and can be fatal. Lactic acid is produced when oxygen levels drop in your body, and a milder form can be a by-product of extreme exercise. It is said to be a cause of the muscle aches you experience the day after a big workout. Symptoms of lactic acidosis include abdominal pain, nausea, and vomiting. Those symptoms are hard to differentiate from the "normal" gastrointestinal side effects of metformin: abdominal pain, diarrhea, nausea, and vomiting.[11] It's worth noting that the "weight loss" drug phenformin was in the same group of medications (biguanides) as metformin but was taken off the market because of severe adverse effects, including lactic acidosis. Brand names of metformin include Glucophage, Glumetza, Fortamet, and Riomet.

Sulfonylureas fight rising blood sugar by squeezing more insulin out of your pancreas. Inherently, these medications work for a short time before they ultimately exhaust your pancreas.[12] Sulfonylureas have more adverse effects and higher mortality rates than metformin, but this medication is also given to patients with more advanced diabetes. Sulfonylureas tend to lower your A1c by less than 1 to 2 percent.[13] That means, for example, that you could expect your A1c to drop from 8.0 to 7.84, which is very little improvement. This medication has been found to exhaust your already weak insulin-producing beta cells and promote weight gain (exactly the opposite of what most diabetics need). Brand names include Dymelor, Glucidoral, Diabenese, Tolinase, and Orinase.

Alpha-glucosidase inhibitors prevent the fast intake of sugar into your blood-stream from your gastrointestinal tract. Because sugar absorption begins in your mouth, there is no way to completely block sugar from entering your bloodstream. For people taking these drugs, the absorption is delayed and sugar is released at a rate that mimics normal digestion. With this drug family, you will still need the insulin secretion from your pancreas to lower your blood sugars, which is why alpha-glucosidase inhibitors work only in the early stages of type 2 diabetes. Later, when the pancreas is exhausted and becomes insulin-deficient, the delay of inflowing sugars provided by this type of medicine makes no difference. The brand names are Glyset and Precose.

The medicinal mushroom maitake functions as a natural alpha-glucosidase inhibitor by preventing the breakdown of sugars and starches without the unwanted side effects from the drugs: flatulence, bloating, belching, and diarrhea.

Dipeptidyl peptidase-4 inhibitors (DPP-4 inhibitors) are newer agents that lower the protein hormone glucagon (which raises blood sugar) by slowing digestion. Since those with diabetes often suffer from a sluggish stomach anyway, this medication can exacerbate that problem. DPP-4 inhibitors tend to be associated with hypoglycemic episodes, lactic acidosis, headaches, and increased infection rates. They also do not aid in weight loss. This medication lowers your A1c by only 1 percent or less. DPP-4 inhibitors are usually recommended in combination with metformin and sulfonylureas. Brand names include Galvus, Januvia, Onglyza, and Tradjenta.

Thiazolidinediones, also known as glytazones, target the DNA of several genes to increase performance at different levels, so they theoretically have several good effects, such as reducing insulin and leptin resistance, hindering the maturing of fat cells, and reducing certain inflammatory markers. Unfortunately, thiazolidinediones typically reduce the A1c by only 2 percent.[14] This group of medications has three members: rosiglytazone (Avandia), troglytazone (Rezulin), and pioglytazone (Actos). Those taking Avandia face increased cardiovascular risks, while those who took Rezulin, which has long since vanished from the market, had an increased risk of liver failure. Actos is still sold in the United States because it compares favorably with the other two in the heart and liver departments. Unfortunately, it has been linked to bladder tumors and has, therefore, been banned in several foreign countries.

Insulin is discussed last because it often is given as the last resort due to its many drawbacks. But insulin has one great advantage over all the other medications: It offers more individual dosage than any of the other anti-diabetic medications. The type of insulin you take (long-acting or short-acting) can be adjusted to your diet and to your blood sugar level.

Insulin comes only as an injection, and many people who have recently been diagnosed with diabetes are living in fear that one day they will have to "take the needle." This drug has been found to promote weight gain, increased appetite, and hypoglycemic episodes.[15-17] Giving an overweight person a drug that leads to weight gain seems counterproductive, but once the pancreas becomes exhausted, there may be no other choice.

Medication versus Lifestyle Intervention

There are good and bad ways to heal. Rather than taking pills and insulin shots, I believe it is better to use your body the way it was intended by Nature in order to heal. And Natural Medicine does this. You may wonder how Natural Medicine differs from other kinds of medicine, such as allopathy (conventional medicine), naturopathy (using naturally occurring substances), and homeopathy (claiming that minute amounts of substances can cure diseases). All of those systems—except for Natural Medicine—rely on using pills as a means of healing. Of course, there is nothing inherently wrong with taking pills. And in certain situations, we need them. But they are vastly overrated and overprescribed, and they can, at times, do more harm than good. Mainly, however, they never address the root cause of the problem: an unhealthy lifestyle. So it should not amaze us that type 2 diabetes responds better to lifestyle changes than to pills and injections.[18-19] My main goal is to help you improve your lifestyle to reverse your diabetes and make your pills unnecessary so you can avoid all of the complications that can result from your medication.

The Diabetic Consequences of Chronic Inflammation

If left to smolder in your body, the same inflammation that caused your diabetes may also cause many other afflictions and diseases including cancer, arthritis, depression, dementia, blindness, amputations, impotence, kidney failure, complications during pregnancy, peripheral vascular disease, polyneuropathy, and increased susceptibility to all kinds of infections.[20-30] And this list doesn't even include all of the little annoyances people with diabetes experience, such as recurrent urinary tract infections, boils, dry and itchy skin, cellulite, blurred vision, tooth and gum infections, fungal infections like athlete's foot, vaginal dryness, gastroparesis, Dupuytren's contracture, and Peyronie's disease.[31-41]

While all of these conditions are worrisome, I believe the extreme exhaustion and voracious, unquenchable hunger people with diabetes experience on a regular basis are the two most pressing issues in their lives. Forget experiencing love, romance, accomplishments, achievements, and being a good parent: Merely surviving every day is a huge effort because hunger and fatigue shorten the day for those afflicted. I believe that hunger functions as a similar signal to pain: Just as pain signals that something is wrong in our bodies, hunger reminds us that we need to eat. In the past, hunger was a serious threat because food was always in short supply. But in these modern times, with our overabundance of food, starvation is unlikely. Instead of worrying about finding food, it's important to try to determine the underlying problem: Why are you feeling hunger in the face of abundance? And how can you fight this extreme fatigue you're experiencing every day? If we want to tackle diabetes, and its root cause, we must address these two debilitating problems first.

Diabetes:
A Low-Energy State

Most men live lives of quiet desperation.

—HENRY DAVID THOREAU (1817–1862)

People with diabetes suffer from a profound fatigue, and it has been my patients' most common complaint. When I asked how they tried to fight this fatigue, most of them responded by telling me that eating junk food was the only thing that provided relief. But that relief lasted only for a short while before the fatigue would return. Then they would have to eat yet again.

People dealing with diabetes often eat just to keep up their energy and to overcome lethargy, a foggy brain, and weariness in each and every limb. And because they have the same everyday responsibilities we all face, like going to work and taking care of their homes and families, they are constantly in a race to eat simply so they can function. It's a vicious cycle stemming from the effect that inflammation has on our bodies. As we discussed in Chapter 1, chronic inflammation causes so much damage in the body that it's not surprising to learn how having diabetes also affects your mitochondria by reducing their energy output.[1] It's as if inflammation stacks wood around the mitochondrial stove until that stove, buried under fuel that can't be reached, is unable to function any longer.

Fatigue and Your Metabolism

Paradoxically, all the food people with diabetes eat to fight fatigue hinders proper metabolism. And each heavy meal only leaves the person weaker, pushing her further down the precipice toward full-blown diabetes-related illnesses. All of that stoked wood becomes a fire hazard: At any moment, the overloaded cell with its buried energy factory can "blow up" into a

How Mitochondria Produce Energy

A mitochondrion is a small organelle inside a cell. Under the electron microscope, it looks a bit like a kid's striped football. It has its own membrane and is a world unto its own inside the cell.

Originally, mitochondria were bacteria taken up into the cell. The cell benefited from the energy the bacterium provided, while the bacterium benefited from the protection of the cell. Meanwhile, the cell and the bacterium (mitochondrion) have lived together for such a long time that each could not live without the other anymore (a state called *symbiosis*).

While the main function of mitochondria is to produce energy, they are also involved in many other functions such as aging, signaling from cell to cell, cell cycle regulation, cell growth, and cell death. And they play an important role in developing insulin resistance.[2] Some cells contain only a single mitochondrion while others contain hundreds or more. Because a mitochondrion was once an intruder, it carries its own private DNA with it.

At any minute in the day, our energy needs can change, like when we go from resting to running or from fasting to gorging. In order to gain extra energy, our mitochondria must produce it by using oxygen to convert glucose and fat into energy storage called adenosine-5-triphosphate (ATP) through a process called aerobic respiration. ATP carries little energy packages and releases them when we need the extra energy. Think of mitochondria as rechargeable batteries: Once your "battery" is charged, you have the energy you need to complete the task at hand.

Energy in mitochondria can be generated anaerobically, as well. But it doesn't astonish me that one way of reloading is *aerobic* respiration. Simply taking in a few deep breaths or performing a little exercise restores our energy. And what's the common thread? Both bring more oxygen into our bodies.

catastrophic illness like a heart attack, a stroke, or an overwhelming infection.

Because diabetics are often lacking energy, their physical and mental abilities can be taxed easily. They scramble to make it through their daily activities and become so exhausted that they usually prefer sleeping or remaining sedentary by sitting on the couch and staring into space or watching television. Watching TV is usually preferred over sitting quietly because their exhaustion is often accompanied by a dreaded sense of failure and despair: Those with diabetes often feel useless and ineffective, and watching TV takes their minds off of this depression.[3]

Part of the depression can be traced back to inflammation in the diabetic brain.[4] For each individual, their low mood is a mixture of factors, perhaps also stemming from constant exhaustion and dealing with the social stigma of being overweight. To preserve energy, diabetics tend to cut down on social interactions, which only fuels the cycle. Without friends and fun, they move even less, further diminishing their metabolic state.

Eliminating Fatigue

So what can be done? We know of two ways to bring mitochondria back to working order: by giving your cells the right amount of the natural, anti-inflammatory foods (fuel) they need and by providing aerobic respiration through exercise. Neither needs to be dreary or unbearable, but because people with diabetes suffer from a constant low-energy state, trying to incorporate even light exercise may seem daunting, and perhaps even unnatural. But diabetes is a genetic affliction that only emerges from living the wrong lifestyle, so patients have only one chance for improvement: to force so-called "unnatural" changes on themselves, against their inclination.

It's important to note that mastering your appetite is not "unnatural"—it only seems that way in a society where food is available 24 hours a day, where people munch on the streets and in their cars, where social gatherings revolve mostly around food, where cookbooks are bestsellers but fewer people can cook than ever before, and where kitchens are expensively renovated but used only for microwaving take-out fare. Our constant heaping up and gobbling down and our way of thinking about food are unnatural. Unfortunately, for the time being, medicine cannot decrease appetites without adverse effects; the pill that takes away those large desires has not yet been invented.

So, this needs to be done: Take a deep breath and choose to eliminate your fatigue. Imagine feeling lighter, healthier, happier, and more energetic. Imagine not depending on food in order to "make it through the day," but instead actually enjoying your activities—and even having energy left over at the end of each day! It's possible to master your appetite and regain your liveliness. But in order to do so, you must first learn more about the obstacles that could hinder your progress. Because it is only when you learn the deep reasons behind why you eat too much (and too often) that you can begin to control your appetite and, ultimately, your fatigue.

Diabetes:
A Voracious State

Let food be thy medicine
and medicine be thy food.

—HIPPOCRATES (C. 460–C. 377 BC)

Diabetes arises from the inflammation inside your body, which primarily takes place in your belly. You already know that belly fat is a direct result of overeating. And you know that this fat—along with the inflammation in your belly—makes you want to eat and eat. But here's a secret: You may not actually be hungry! In the previous chapter, we described diabetes as a *low-energy state* because it saps you of all strength. Now let's talk about its *voracious* aspect.

Why do people with type 2 diabetes and prediabetes overeat? Is it entirely their fault? No, this overeating is a direct result of our modern lives, for which our ancient bodies are inherently unfit. The food industry pushes inferior foods down our throats. Even our government is to blame, with their unwholesome food pyramid based on white starches and dairy.

Another problem? Conventional medicine manages diabetes, but doesn't cure it. A recent study showed that screening once for diabetes and giving the diagnosis doesn't improve the outcome for the patient.[1] So what does this mean? Simply giving a diagnosis is not enough! This diagnosis doesn't teach you how to reverse the chronic inflammation in your body, cure your diabetes,

37

or even fight the hunger that caused your problem in the first place. But sometimes a patient is desperate for a diagnosis—any diagnosis. If she has been going from doctor to doctor and has been told multiple times that nothing is wrong and it's all in her head, she might be relieved to finally be told she has chronic fatigue or some other syndrome. Now she knows what ails her, so she can tell her family and her boss. Now she can finally deal with it.

Sometimes a diagnosis can save a life: If your belly hurts and the diagnosis is appendicitis, a surgeon will operate on you and your life will be saved. Sometimes, however, a diagnosis is just a word. If your doctor tells you that you have hypertension, or high blood pressure, that doesn't help you very much. It does, however, help the doctor decide what pill to prescribe you— for the rest of your life. Now you are a patient.

The uncomfortable truth is that health does not come from a bottle of pills. Specific lifestyle advice and implementation is required. What *you* decide to do with your life determines your health. The conventional view of diabetes is that it is a disease of too much sugar in the blood. The medications you're prescribed, therefore, use different mechanisms to lower blood sugar levels. But do they ever address your insatiable hunger—the root of your condition?

How Hungry Are You—**Really?**

Science has shown that there is more to diabetes than just having elevated blood sugar.[2] Chronic inflammation is at the root, and it affects fat, sugar, energy metabolism, and immune function, along with every cell in your body. But from the patient's perspective, diabetes feels like constant exhaustion and hunger: Diabetics' appetites are insatiable, and as a result, about 90 percent are overweight.[3] One researcher has termed this kind of *misplaced* hunger as the Empty Hollow Sensation (EHS).[4] But even in light of the horrible consequences of diabetes, people with diabetes can't stop eating, and food is on their minds constantly. So how do you tackle the biggest hurdle diabetics face? How can you stop thinking about food and overcome this Empty Hollow Sensation? By becoming aware of the different factors fueling your limitless appetite, you may begin to conquer the cravings that led to your inflammation—and ultimately, your diabetes.

Are You Really Hungry, **or Are You Just Emptying Your Plate Like a "Good Girl"?**

Did your parents encourage you to empty your plate as a child? In the past, being thin was a threat to many children's lives and, therefore, a worry for parents. Tuberculosis, for instance, is less likely to strike a chubby child and was most likely the reason your parents and grandparents urged you to clean your plate. But you are no longer a child, and these days, we have the opposite problem: obesity. So stop cleaning your plate like a "good girl," or serve yourself smaller portions! Start listening to your body when it sends signals of fullness. And never, ever take a second helping!

Are You Really Hungry, **or Are You Just Thirsty?**

When your body tries to communicate, you may understand so little of its language that you think you are hungry when, in reality, you are thirsty. This is a common misinterpretation, and it's a major issue for people with diabetes, who tend to be thirstier than others because elevated blood sugar increases thirst. Physiologically, we confuse hunger with thirst because they both are regulated in the same part of our brain, the hypothalamus.[5]

So if you can't rely on your hunger and thirst sensations, how do you tell the difference? Drink a cup of warm water or herbal tea. After a few moments, ask yourself if you are still hungry. Often, you will find that your hunger has disappeared. It's also worth noting that once you reach age 50, the functionality of the thirst center in your brain begins to decline, even in those who don't have diabetes.[6] You will have to learn how to gauge your own water needs and remind yourself to drink the amount of water you require each day. (We'll talk about this more in Chapter 11.)

Are You Really Hungry, **or Are You Seduced by Advertisements?**

Certain foods, like corn, wheat, and dairy, are subsidized by the government. The food industry uses these cheap ingredients to manufacture snack foods that sound delicious in advertisements. These cheap ingredients also appeal to manufacturers for another reason: Salt, sugar, and hydrogenated fats give products a long shelf life.

Think for a moment: Do you ever see advertisements for apples or a head of cabbage? No. Yet apples and cabbage do wonders for your health, whereas boxed cereal or a new power drink will undermine it.

You can listen to your body signaling hunger or satiety—or you can listen to food manufacturers bidding to entice you to overeat "yummy" processed foods. Advertisers spend about $10 billion on food advertisements each year.[7] Do you think they do this to promote good health? No; they address you as a shopper and only want your money. Consider them to be enablers of the obesity and diabetes epidemics in this country. Meanwhile, learn to decipher the deceiving language manufacturers use to entice you into buying their food products in "How to Read Labels" on page 108.

Are You Really Hungry, or Are You Hypoglycemic?

What happens when you skip a meal? Do you become weak, sweaty, and grouchy if you go too long without eating? Does your brain stop working until you get another doughnut into your system? And will the same hunger, irritability, and shaking recur a few hours later? If so, you may be experiencing *hypoglycemia*, and not hunger.

Hypoglycemia means low blood sugar. If you eat simple carbohydrates like sugars and starches, your blood glucose will spike quickly because those simple sugars are so easily digested. And since digestion actually starts in your mouth and not your stomach, that sugar is immediately absorbed into your body.

As we learned in Chapter 2, a spike in blood sugar is a state of emergency because high blood sugar is toxic for cells. In this emergency, your pancreas releases large amounts of insulin to lower your blood sugar. Your insulin output usually is too high for that sugar spike, which lowers your blood sugar too much, and 2 or 3 hours later, you will find yourself in the midst of the next emergency: hypoglycemia.

This constant overtaxing of your pancreas is one mechanism that leads to type 2 diabetes—your pancreas becomes exhausted and slowly gives up. The second mechanism, of course, is that your cells, tired of always being rushed into emergency response, become insulin resistant. They don't adequately answer to your body screaming "fire!" any longer.

Here is how to tell whether you are prone to bouts of hypoglycemia: Can you skip a meal? If you can, you probably don't need to worry about hypoglycemia. A well-fed (and I don't mean overweight) person can go for several hours without feeling the need to eat. You will learn more tricks later, but if you stick to the harvest of Earth—greens, roots, fruits, nuts, legumes, and whole grains—you will slowly get plenty of fuel for your cells. A slow release of sugar is what our bodies are designed for, not for the sudden rush and high of modern junk.

Are You Really Hungry, or Are You Just a Creature of Habit?

When the clock strikes noon, what's your first thought? Odds are, you begin thinking about lunch. But what if you had a late breakfast and aren't hungry? Do you listen to your body, or do you eat another meal simply because it's "lunchtime"?

We often associate specific times of day or events with food. Think about birthday parties, social business gatherings, and Sundays after church: All of these scenarios typically include food—but we're missing the point of these gatherings. It took me a while to believe that I am not a bad hostess at my writers' group meetings if I don't offer something to eat. I used to put nuts and dried fruit on the table until we decided that tea was sufficient. After all, we don't need to munch while we're working. And when we celebrate, we should focus on people, not food.

Don't eat just because it is time to eat, or because you have nothing else to do. Unnecessary eating can hinder your progress as you try to fight the inflammation in your body, so try to find new ways to spend your time. Instead of focusing on food, take up a new fun hobby, or maybe even spend some time as a volunteer. By learning good habits, you won't have time to miss that extra food you were eating.

Are You Really Hungry, or Are You Devouring One Mammoth after the Other?

This is the paradox: The more you eat, the more weight you gain—and the more famished you feel! In olden times, when food was scarce, this was a survival instrument: If a whole mammoth had to be devoured before it spoiled, people needed to be able to gorge themselves beyond the point of feeling full. This allowed them to put on fat for leaner times. And those leaner times always came. But these days, they never come. Yet we still feel the need to eat as much as we can.

Contrary to what seems obvious (namely that an overweight person would seem to be blissfully satisfied and easily able to cut down on calorie intake), many who are overweight never feel satisfied. An ancient survival tool makes them feel extremely hungry and forces them to eat even more. As a rule of thumb, the slimmer you are, the less hunger you feel. The larger you are, the more ravenous you become.

People who are overweight tend to suffer from incredible hunger pangs, which are largely not acknowledged by the medical community or are chalked up to "a lack of willpower." You can identify this hunger by paying special attention to your cravings: Does your hunger strike at the sight of food? If so, odds are that this "mammoth" hunger is what you're experiencing.

Are You Really Hungry, or Do You Have an Underactive Thyroid?

A sluggish thyroid makes you gain weight in two ways: You feel constant hunger, and you are too lethargic to move much. If you are overweight, have your thyroid levels tested; an underactive thyroid could be the underlying cause. In addition to weight gain and fatigue, other signs of a sluggish thyroid include constipation, a slow heart beat, excessive sleepiness, feeling cold all the time, thinning hair, and dry skin. If your doctor determines that you have an underactive thyroid, have her test your tolerance for gluten, as well. Hypothyroidism and gluten intolerance are often linked: Gluten creates inflammation, and this inflammation hits the thyroid and burns it out.

Are You Really Hungry, or Are You Imprinted by What Your Mother Ate during Pregnancy?

Did you know that babies in utero swallow and taste? If mothers eat foods like garlic and carrots during pregnancy, the food flavors show up in the amniotic fluid around the growing baby, giving the baby a taste of what the mother eats. And the baby later forms preferences for food that he or she already "knows."[8]

Research also links part of the obesity epidemic in children (and grown-ups) to mothers who were overweight and diabetic. But studies on children of survivors of the famine during World War II in Europe have shown that underfed mothers can also breed obese, diabetic children. What these two divergent situations teach us is that any deviation from an ideal weight can lead to weight complications in the next generation.

Fathers have an impact, too: Studies show that what a man eats during sperm production influences the weight and health of his future offspring.[9] Sperm are produced constantly, so the time for men to think about healthy eating is *before* they are ready to become fathers.

If both of your parents are overweight, you have three factors contributing to your insatiable appetite: Genes from your mother, genes from your father, and, in all likelihood, an environment that furthers mindless eating. But you can break this cycle by choosing to eat a well-rounded anti-inflammatory diet now, so you can pass along healthier genes to future generations.

Are You Really Hungry, or Are You Sleep Deprived and Stressed?

Have you ever searched through your house for something to eat—opening and closing the fridge door or rummaging through the pantry—while still trying to be "good" and stay on your diet? Have you ever considered that you might not be hungry but *tired*, instead?

Studies tie your hunger to the *ghrelin* hormone, levels of which rise when you are sleep deprived.[10] I call ghrelin the "growling and prowling hormone" because it makes you cranky, voracious, clumsy, and ineffective. Sleep deprivation and stress both elevate your ghrelin levels, making you ravenous. And the foods you crave are typically high in sugar, bad fats, and calories—all of which increase inflammation and make you more prone to developing diabetes.[11]

When we sleep, we fast because our bodies stop sending hunger signals, which would disturb our sleep. So, if you don't give in to your urge to eat late or in the middle of the night and you sleep, instead, your system returns your ghrelin levels back to normal—and your hunger disappears![12] Studies have shown that your circadian rhythm (your internal clock) is linked to your genes. Some people are night owls and some are morning people, while most fall somewhere in the middle. Interestingly, the night owls in the study got less sleep, had higher ghrelin levels, and tended to be overweight.[13]

So, while you may be stuck with your night owl genes, you can choose to change your habits. Try to go to bed earlier at night, and keep track of any changes in your hunger levels. You will likely find that your late-night snacking habits are no longer a problem.

Are You Really Hungry, or Are You Fighting Your Circadian Rhythm?

It is true that people are eating the *wrong* foods. But a bigger problem is that food is constantly offered. As a culture, we teach our children that it is always time to eat. When a child shows up in the kitchen outside of mealtimes, we ask: "Are you hungry, sweetie?" When the child is sad or bored, we offer cookies. There is a constant need to be fed, to be entertained, to be rewarded, to be cajoled, to be kept quiet—and it seems that food is always involved.

If you're constantly eating, your body is always busy with digestion and has no time for the repair and rebuilding we discussed in Chapter 1. As a result, your inner clock, or circadian rhythm, gets out of balance and you cannot function well, sleep well, think well, or live well.

Natural Medicine has long stressed the importance of getting enough sleep, regular sleep patterns, and good sleeping habits. The convenience of electricity has changed the world profoundly, but it hasn't made a dent in our ancient bodies and primordial souls: They still have the same physiological and emotional needs that they've always had. Yes, you can raid the fridge in the middle of the night, go shopping in the wee hours, or sit at your computer all night long—but in the long run, going against your natural sleep-wake cycle will take a toll on your body. Keep the time between dinner and breakfast for fasting, and give your body a chance to rest and repair.

Are You Really Hungry, or Has Yo-Yo Dieting Destroyed Your Confidence?

Your body is a wonderful machinery of precise checks and balances. Sure, right now with your diabetes, your system seems out of balance, but your body still has the ability to heal. Losing weight, regaining weight, losing weight, and regaining some more sends confusing signals to your body, not to mention your brain, which is responsible for steering this machinery.

A recent study refuted the claim that *yo-yo dieting*, or *weight cycling*—those ups and downs of your waist and weight—has a negative impact on your ability to lose weight in the future.[14] What the study does not take into account, however, is how discouraging it is to regain, time after time, what you have lost with such great effort. You lose heart.

You can only begin to heal your body by learning what drove the fast loss/ slow regain cycle. Successful weight loss consists of losing the weight and *keeping* it off. Don't believe anybody who promises you quick results, because those results won't last. Instead, follow The Five Health Essentials in Part 3 (see page 77) to reverse your diabetes and regain your health. This time, you'll lose those extra pounds for good because you'll be relying on the healing power of Nature and not on your willpower alone.

Are You Really Hungry, or Is Your Competitive Drive Focused on Food?

Some people are not hungry, but they need to grab the biggest piece of the pie anyway. Are you one of them? This often stems from sibling rivalry and too much hardship growing up. Try cutting back on your portions a little, so that the biggest piece of pie does not always land on your hips!

Are You Really Hungry, or Are You Struggling to Overcome Childhood Trauma?

Throughout my career as a physician, I have often found that many overeaters are struggling to overcome a traumatic childhood experience—typically abuse. If this rings true for you, continue reading. Otherwise, feel free to skip ahead to the next topic.

Victims of childhood abuse often feel helpless and find that eating or gaining weight grants them a certain amount of power and protection. And while this applies to victims of all kinds of abuse (physical, mental, verbal, and sexual), I've found that sexual abuse victims are generally more susceptible to overeating, and as a result are at an increased risk for developing obesity and diabetes. About 30 percent of females have a history of childhood sexual abuse; males have half that number. And subsequent health issues loom large for both sexes.

If needed, work up your old history with an experienced counselor. Don't continue to waste more minutes of your precious life feeling unhappy, wounded, and unfulfilled! If you feel the need to eat when you're not actually hungry, try writing in a journal. By turning to this therapeutic practice, not only will you finally address your struggles from childhood, but you'll also begin to remove your dependence on food.

Signs You May Have a Food Allergy

- **Fatigue.** You grow tired after each meal. We all are tired after a heavy meal, but if you are extremely tired even after a smaller meal, you may have a food allergy.

- **Abdominal discomfort.** This typically occurs within minutes of finishing a meal, but unfortunately it can even take a day or two. Your stomach may feel bloated and distended. Diarrhea is a more severe sign and, if chronic or intermittently recurrent, should be evaluated by a physician. Heartburn is seldom recognized as stemming from food allergies, but it often goes away when you stop eating nightshades (tomatoes, bell peppers, chile peppers, eggplants, and potatoes), nuts, or dairy.

- **Weakness.** Try lifting your arms 15 minutes after you finish a meal. If they feel heavy or ache more than usual (compared to how light you felt in the morning), you may have a food allergy.

- **Musculoskeletal system aches.** Joint, tendon, and muscle problems can all be warning signs. If you experience aches or problems such as bursitis, try eliminating nuts and dairy. You may also want to get evaluated for celiac disease (gluten intolerance).

- **Mouth problems.** A burning sensation in your mouth, an aching palate, tickling in your throat, or sores inside your mouth or on your tongue might signal an allergy.

Are You Really Hungry,
or Are You Addicted to Your Food?

You suspected as much: Your eating habits might be an addiction. *Liking* a food is different from *craving* a food. By linking ordinary food with pleasurable activities, you went from merely enjoying a food to feeling like you can't live without it. Or there may be something in your food (such as endorphin-like substances in grains) that makes you want more and more. Cravings for fat or protein are rare; people typically crave simple carbohydrates. It is not

- **Bladder issues.** Slow urine flow can be a sign of a food allergy, due to a swelling of the urethra. Recurrent urinary tract infections, with or without bacteria growing out in culture or burning in the urethra (in males), are also warning signs. An irritable bladder (interstitial cystitis) may respond to eliminating coffee and certain foods.

- **Thirst.** If you are thirstier than other people—always running around with a water bottle in your hand—think *allergy.* If you get thirsty right after a meal or you drink much more than your peers, you may be thirsty because your body wants to flush out what it perceives to be a toxin: the allergen. If you drink, you dilute the dangerous substance in your blood, and it becomes less damaging.

- **Other symptoms.** The following diseases and complaints have also been linked to food allergies: headaches, asthma, swollen glands, bleeding and inflamed gums, abdominal discomfort and bloating, diarrhea, itchy skin, recurrent infections (sinus, UTI, etc.), itchy eyes, listlessness and mild depression, obesity and bulimia, recurrent phlebitis, anal itching and/or rashes, low blood pressure, dizziness, and breast pain. Consult with your doctor if you're experiencing any of the symptoms above, since all of these conditions may also be symptoms of a serious illness.

by chance that gluten sensitivity and alcoholism (and type 2 diabetes!) are linked by addictive behavior and the dopamine pathway. By rotating and alternating your foods, you will not only avoid addiction to certain foods, but you will also be able to avoid certain food allergies.

Are You Really Hungry, or Are Your Allergies Making You Crave Forbidden Foods?

Every time a patient tells me, "I just *love* ice cream!" (or cheese, or whatever) I say, "You shouldn't love food—you should love your mate!" Every time you find yourself saying you "love" something edible, start reexamining your eating habits—and your life.

People who "love" certain foods often have an allergy to those foods. The mechanism is unclear, but the foods to which we're allergic are often the very foods we eat on a regular basis. And the reason why we eat them so often is because we associate those foods with pleasure or a reward.[15]

One shouldn't "love" cheese, and yet, so many people do. Very often, the beloved food is from the dairy group or is loaded with sugar and artificial molecules. (My downfall is whipped cream or sour cream—the fattier, the better!) But these are the very foods that cause your body to increase zonulin, a recently discovered protein that modulates how tightly the cells in the bowel are connected. When zonulin is increased, the tight junctions between your gut cells loosen, increasing the likelihood that food particles will fall through these "holes" and come into contact with your blood. (This condition is called *leaky gut syndrome*.) In turn, your body mounts antibodies against those food particles, and with that, you have developed a new food allergy. But while you may still crave those "forbidden" foods, you can no longer eat them because once you have an allergy, eating more of that food will worsen the leaky gut.[16]

I used to eat nuts daily, until I realized they caused my extreme fatigue. But no food should appear on your menu every single day. You can decrease your chances of developing a food allergy simply by incorporating more variety into your diet.[17] And if you suspect that a specific type of food is harming your body, see Chapter 7 to learn how to replace it with foods that will lower the inflammation in your body.

Any food can become a culprit. If you have pinpointed one food item as allergenic for you, compare it with other items in the same botanical family.

Rick's Story

Compared to the "normal" hefty American male, Rick was just a wisp of a guy: 145 pounds at 5 feet 10 inches. When he consulted with me, his hemoglobin A1c was 5.8, which meant he was prediabetic. For a "natural" physician like me, this was cause for (mild) alarm. Sure, he had a bit of a belly. But his diet was extremely good: He happened to like vegetables, and his wife cooked them daily. Among my patients, Rick had one of the healthiest diets: He had only fruit for breakfast, salads for lunch, and vegetables with fish or meat for dinner. And he never snacked—except at 11:00 p.m.

Rick was an engineer, and in the evening he would pore over the numbers on his computer until he would finally shut down his laptop and relax. He told me that when all of his work was done, he rewarded himself with a shot of whiskey and a good handful of nuts, raisins, dried fruit, and chocolate. I did not begrudge him this little indulgence, but I told him that his body needed the time between 11:00 p.m. and 1:00 a.m. for repair. If his stomach was busy digesting, the repair would be compromised.

Rick had no intention of listening to me—and he didn't, for several years. One day he returned to my office with a bad case of psoriasis, which began while he was traveling and indulged in a new trail mix. I immediately suspected a nut allergy. He also had eaten more cheese on the road than his wife allowed at home. He tested positive for allergies to dairy, nuts, soy, and balm of Peru (a fragrance used in many cosmetics).

Reluctantly, Rick omitted his evening snack, and to his surprise, he lost 5 pounds. He had never thought of himself as overweight, but his small belly disappeared. At his next visit, his A1c had dropped from 5.8 to 5.2. By simply removing the offending food from his diet, Rick had eliminated the allergy-induced inflammation that caused his prediabetes. He was now out of the diabetes danger zone. He did not have to give up his chocolate indulgence for good. Instead, Rick changed to a dark, milk-free variety and ate it during the day, instead of at night. His psoriasis healed nicely, and he was proud to have shed that little belly of his.

For example, if you react poorly to apples, you might react to pears; if you have an allergic response to cherries, you may also have a reaction to peaches, plums, and apricots.

Every allergy-inducing food acts like an inflammatory agent in your body.[18] Nuts, for instance, are a near-perfect food, with their anti-inflammatory omega-3 fatty acids and abundance of good minerals. But once you have a nut allergy, they are your enemy food.

Are You Really Hungry, **or Are You Bored?**

Does it seem like you have nothing better to do than eat? Eating out of boredom is a huge danger sign that you might never get out of your diabetic condition because you need it: You need to eat to keep yourself entertained, and you need the diabetes diagnosis so you can tell your boss, your friends, and your family that you have a *real* disease.

Is it your arthritis that keeps you from going to interesting places? Are you married to your insulin syringe? Are you relieved to have an excuse not to work? Is your doctor's appointment as exciting as a rendezvous? Do you find yourself constantly thinking or talking about your ailments? Those all are danger signs.

Instead of succumbing to your diagnosis, fight it by keeping yourself busy and trying something new. If you're occupied by something else, you're less likely to overeat due to boredom.

Are You Really Hungry, **or Do You Just Feel the Need to Eat Something Crunchy?**

We eat so many soft foods—breads, cheeses, burgers, tomatoes, pasta, pizza, lasagna, meatballs—that we often crave something hard to grind between our molars.[19] Food manufacturers know that crunchy food is an easy sale; potato chips prove that point. Go back to eating naturally crunchy foods like nuts and apples, which don't hurt your metabolism and still satisfy the needs of the masticatory machinery of your mouth. (Bonus: Using chewing muscles will tone your facial features!)

As it turns out, soft food is also often *white*, doubling the injury to your body because color in food signals that it contains antioxidants and other polyphenols. White foods (like sugar, starches, and Wonder Bread) are often overly processed and contain none of the wonderfully invigorating plant compounds that quench the inflammation in your body.

Colorful Food

A simple way to know that you're choosing natural, healthy food is to focus on eating colorful food. Each color in Nature has distinct health benefits, so refer to this list to learn what you can expect to get from your food based on its natural color.

- **Green:** Chlorophyll and glucosinolates give green foods their color. Consumed alone, glucosinolates may be bitter, but in your diet, you can't get enough of them: They are the sulfur compounds in most cabbages. You know that greens are healthy for you: Green bell peppers, broccoli, chard, collard greens, dandelion, dinosaur kale, kale, and herbs all keep your immune system healthy and promote digestion and circulation.

- **Red:** Carotenoids and flavonoids (including lycopene) lure you with reddish colors. Red looks enticing—but also alarming. Red foods like apples and red cherries catch your eye, but the color red also has another connotation. If you see a red berry on a bush that you don't know, it sounds an alarm: Could it be poisonous? Red foods catch free radicals before they damage your cells. They mainly affect the health of your blood vessels, and they do it by lowering oxidative stress, helping with cell repair, and decreasing inflammation.[20] Red foods you should enjoy include red peppers, tomatoes, red currants, red beets, rosehips, pink grapefruit, cherries, red chard, and strawberries.

- **Blue:** Nature doesn't give us a true blue in food—it would signal death and spoilage. But it gives us blue antioxidants like indole and anthocyanins, which are often underlined with red flavonoids so that the result is purple. Examples include blueberries, eggplants, red cabbage, plums, prunes, and forbidden (black) rice. Anthocyanins are good for our immune systems. They lower cholesterol, balance female and male hormones, and douse inflammation.

- **Yellow:** Yellow's spectrum goes from greenish yellow (lutein) to orangey yellow (flavonoids), and we find this color in citrus fruits, pineapple, yellow plums, August apples, summer squash, and yellow bell peppers.

- **Orange:** Carrots get their color from carotenes, which promote eye health, as do sweet potatoes, melons, and chanterelles.

Are You Really Hungry, or Are You Just Frustrated and Upset?

The other day I had an upsetting exchange with a couple in the parking lot of the supermarket. The man claimed that I had done damage to his car; I had not. Now, nothing really happened—it was a minor case of road rage. But when I arrived home, I was shaking. I had kept my cool in front of the couple, but at home I broke down, and I made myself a bowl of muesli with soymilk—knowing full well that they are not the best foods for my joints and my stomach, but comfort food was what I craved. And yes, it calmed me down and made me happy, and this incident was an exception to my typical dietary choices. But what if I needed to eat unhealthy things every single day when I came home from work because my boss overburdens me with last-minute requests? Or what if I turned to ice cream every time my mate yelled at me, or whenever I found the letter box overflowing with unpaid bills?

Comfort food is for rare emergencies. Instead of turning to food, try to determine the psychological reasons why you eat too much. Write those reasons in your journal and start working on your issues. And once in a blue moon, give in to that craving for comforting soul food!

Are You Really Hungry, or Are You Unhappy, Unfulfilled, and Lonely?

There's no doubt that unhappiness makes us eat. But eating does not make us happy, because if you eat the wrong foods—or even the right foods at wrong times—you damage your gut, your brain, and every cell in your body by stoking inflammation. This ultimately destroys your health, which will lead to deeper depression.

Learn to change your mood in a lasting way, and you'll get healthier in the process. Instead of facing your health concerns on your own, connect with your inner self and with people around you (see Chapter 10 for suggestions). If you think you need more help, speak with your physician. But before going on medication for depression, try incorporating small amounts of exercise (see Chapter 9), a good diet, and some gentle herbs like St. John's wort into your diet.

Are You Really Hungry, or Are You Hanging Out with the Wrong Crowd?

Get this: People who live, work, and play together tend to be similar in size. Studies have shown that you are not only what you eat—after a while, you are also like the people around you.[21] So while obesity isn't contagious, the thoughts of your friends, and their eating habits, are!

I'm not saying you should end your important relationships. If you have a friend who is overweight, instead of giving in to her denial and rationalization of her food choices by adopting them for your own, why not gently nudge her to follow your new path toward better health? Tell her how excited you are about the amazing discoveries you have made, and take her on your journey. You can still be her friend, even if she doesn't listen—but get your standards from other people.

Are You Really Hungry, or Are Your Gut Bacteria Sending Weird Messages to Your Brain?

On one level, it is really not *you* craving food, it's the bacteria in your gut! Studies have found that people who are overweight have different bacteria in their guts than those who are lean.[22] So if you are eating the wrong foods— and too much of them—you are feeding bad bacteria. By changing to a healthier diet, you can starve those greedy bacteria to death, better bacteria will grow, and you'll be less hungry.[23]

When we are born, we have no bacteria in our intestines. But within a few hours, bacteria invade and build up their specific environments. The food we provide to an infant determines the kind of bacteria that will grow. For example, if we gave sugar water to an infant right after birth, it would cause different bacteria to grow in his bowels than if he were fed his mother's milk.

So how do your gut and your brain talk to each other? Neurotransmitters— small messenger molecules—are produced by your cells, and also by gut bacteria. Some of your gut bacteria are friendly and beneficial, but others are not. The bad guys are those that are sending "Hunger!" cries to your brain long after you should be satisfied, because they feel threatened if you don't feed them sugars and starches. So, with every good food choice you make, you support the good bacteria and diminish the bad bacteria, which reduces the number of "hungry" signals sent to your brain.

You can also promote good bacteria in your gut by taking probiotics. The belief is that beneficial gut bacteria like *Lactobacillus* and *Bifidobacterium* will repopulate your intestines. Loosely translated, probiotics means "for life," and recent research maintains that probiotics are one of the two most helpful supplements money can buy (the other being fish oil). Side effects may include cramping and occasional diarrhea, so if one strain or brand bothers you, try another. Also, start with a low dose, and slowly increase the amount you take as your bowels get used to it.

It is not completely clear how probiotics work because studies on gut bacteria have shown that it is very hard to change the composition of bacteria in the gut.[24] However, clinical studies have shown that probiotics are useful—especially for leaky gut, allergies, and autoimmune diseases.[25]

Are You Really Hungry, or Is Your White Fat Crying for Food?

Are you an apple or a pear? "Apples" accumulate their surplus calories in fat around their bellies and are prone to diabetes. "Pears" tend to be heavy below the waist (around the thighs) and are less likely to develop diabetes but have a higher propensity for obesity. If you are an "apple," your belly may be carrying your death.

So what is it in your belly that could kill you? Fat. Abdominal fat is dangerous because most of the harmful effects of metabolism happen in belly fat[26]—your white fat, to be precise. We have two kinds of fat: white and brown. Simply stated, brown fat is good fat and white fat is bad fat.

Brown fat behaves less like fat and more like muscle. It is located mostly in the back of your neck and around your shoulders and gets its darker color from mitochondria and their iron content. It has more blood vessels for better oxygenation and is metabolically more active than white fat. And here's some good news: Brown fat actually burns calories instead of storing them, and it helps you lose weight by speeding up your metabolism. It can also decrease insulin resistance.

Belly fat is completely made up of white fat, and it is white fat that keeps the fires of inflammation smoldering.[27] It manufactures all kinds of inflammatory small messenger molecules called cytokines, as well as other signaling peptides (small proteins). One example of these messenger molecules is hormones, which bring signals from your sexual organs to your brain. Those belly fat–derived metabolical hormones are called *adipokines*.

You may think fat is just sitting there, doing nothing but storing your extra calories, but white belly fat is actually one of the main communication centers in your body. It reigns over your hunger and your satiety, your cravings and your dislikes. It rules your metabolism, oversees the development of new small blood vessels, affects lipids in your blood, produces insulin sensitivity, governs bleeding mechanisms, controls your energy balance, and, through various growth factors, may induce cancer development. These adipokines are high in white fat and are responsible for obesity, insulin resistance, and diabetes.

Adipokines from your abdominal fat also send out messages to your brain asking for more food since the fat cells have only one goal: to grow. White belly fat cells grow with the same immodesty as cancer cells. But by taking control of your health and your diabetes, you will begin to diminish this white fat and rebuild your brown, healthy fat.

Are You Really Hungry, or Are Your Cold Mitochondria Promoting Obesity?

Do you know how your body creates heat? There are two ways: One is *shivering thermogenesis*, meaning that if you shiver, your muscles' involuntary oscillations produce heat, preventing you from dying of hypothermia. The second way is *non-shivering thermogenesis*, meaning those oscillations are undetectably taking place inside your cells—in the mitochondria of brown fat.

A heat-producing protein called *thermogenin* (also called *uncoupling protein*, or *PGC-1 alpha*) sits on the inner cell walls of your mitochondria. In order to produce heat, however, your body needs essential fatty acids such as healthy oils.[28] So this process cannot happen if you are on a low-fat or fat-free diet, or if the fats in your food are inferior, like fried oils, rancid oils, margarine, or shortening. Without essential fatty acids, your mitochondria stay cold and don't burn the fat you want to get rid of.[29]

If your mitochondria remain cold, you begin craving fatty foods, and if you don't pay attention, you'll find yourself eating the wrong fatty foods. Healthy fats (olive oil, coconut oil, and ghee) promote non-shivering thermogenesis, which in turn will burn your fat. And exposure to cold—going outside on a cold day, turning down the thermostat in your place, going swimming, taking a cold shower—will aid in building up your brown fat and will ultimately fight hunger.

Are You Really Hungry, or Is Your Diet Suppressing Your Fat-Busting Glucagon Levels?

Glucagon is the counterplayer to insulin: Like insulin, glucagon is a hormone that's manufactured in the pancreas. When your blood sugar is high, insulin levels rise, inhibiting glucagon at the same time. But as soon as blood sugar levels are dangerously low, glucagon kicks in and quickly makes sugar available to your fuel-starved cells.[30] Glucagon gets sugar into your bloodstream fast by binding to receptors on liver cells, which in turn break down the long, starchy chains stored in your liver into single sugar molecules.

Insulin and glucagon make sure your blood sugar levels are not too high (and toxic) or too low, as sugar is the fuel on which most biochemical actions in your body depend. Your brain would be the first to go because it needs the greatest amount of sugar to function. Glucagon also hinders glycogen synthesis, because when sugar is low, every molecule is needed in circulation; to store it at that time would be the wrong move. And here comes the bummer: If you constantly have high blood sugar, your insulin is always high and suppresses glucagon. This means that glucagon cannot work for you and turn your fat deposits into useful energy because you remain dependent on the constant intake of food instead of using your fat stores.

Are You Really Hungry, or Is Your Low Adiponectin Level Reducing Your Energy?

Adiponectin is one of the adipokines produced in the fat cells that works to eliminate fat and increase insulin sensitivity in your cells.[31] But when an increased amount of white fat keeps your body in the low-smoldering inflammation state that eventually leads to the development of diabetes, less adiponectin is released from your overburdened fat cells. So when you need it most, your adiponectin fails, and increased insulin resistance is the consequence. And this is when diabetes begins.

Low adiponectin levels are bad because they mean you burn less fat and don't effectively clear sugar from your blood. Higher adiponectin levels would not only fight the inflammation in your body, but also would curb your hunger.[32] Research also shows that low adiponectin impairs peak performance of the affected muscles. In other words, if you are overweight, your muscles tire more easily because they cannot perform the way they should. The sad part is that your heart is a muscle, too—and low adiponectin also reduces the strength with which your heart beats.[33]

So, what can you do to increase adiponectin and reap its many benefits? Move a little more throughout the day and avoid sugars and starches at dinner. It really is that simple!

Are You Really Hungry, or Is Your Leptin Level Tricking You?

Leptin is known as the satiety hormone; without it, we eat and eat and never feel satisfied.

But leptin does not respond as much to a single meal. Instead, it senses how much fat your body harbors—your overall nutritional status—and rises in direct proportion, decreasing your appetite.

So if leptin rises in accordance with the amount of fat stored in your body, why don't those who are overweight experience satiety? Lack of sleep can be to blame: When you don't get enough rest at night, your leptin levels decrease, and you don't feel satisfied after a meal.[34] At the same time, emotional stress can cause your leptin levels to rise, or to remain constantly high, leading to leptin resistance, which drives you to eat more in order to obtain more energy.[35] But your cells never truly feel satisfied because they can't meet this energy demand, and as a result, they stop responding to the high leptin levels. Once this happens, you've developed *leptin resistance*, which is similar to insulin resistance. It is believed that leptin problems come first, followed by diabetes.[36] And doesn't it make sense? First you experience stress, which leads to overeating, weight gain, and then diabetes. Sounds like the story of our modern times, doesn't it?

Paradoxically, you need those leptin levels to come down so that you get hungry again, eat, and have your high leptin levels signal that you are happily full. But how can you bring those leptin levels down in the first place? Try to lose some weight by cutting sugars and white starches. Eat vegetables to provide your cells with healthy nutrients, and include good fats and a bit of protein in every meal. Chew well and eat slowly: This will give your leptin time to come down. And go to bed early!

Are You Really Hungry, or Does Your Ghrelin Level Make High-Calorie Foods Irresistible?

While leptin is the satiety hormone, ghrelin is the hunger hormone, and it is just as complicated; it rises with sleep deprivation and stress. But there is more to ghrelin: It uses the pleasure centers in your brain and is responsible for cravings for "comfort foods"—basically everything that's sweet and fat. And these cravings typically set in at night.

When it functions properly, ghrelin is low after dinner and slowly rises in the early morning hours, making you hungry in time for breakfast. But ghrelin levels tend to be lower in those who struggle with their weight. People who are stressed and overweight lose the ability to determine whether or not they are hungry, and when that happens, they typically choose to eat.

The best way to fight those "comfort food" cravings is to create a bedtime schedule and stick to it. Just as with leptin, if you're sleeping, you won't feel the hunger. That means you can wake up the next morning and begin to eat on schedule.

Are You Really Hungry, or Are Your High-Calorie, Nutrient-Depleted Foods Leaving Your Cells Crying for More?

So much of our food is inferior to what our ancestors ate in the past. Food is now grown in depleted soil (destroyed by artificial fertilizers and pesticides), stored for extended times, and adulterated to a degree that our cells can't even recognize it as food. Laced with artificial colors, artificial flavors, and artificial preservatives, the "foods" you shove into your mouth on a daily basis aren't really foods at all. And all of these empty calories leave your body deprived of vitamins, antioxidants, and polyphenols, which causes your cells to cry out for more food. You may be overweight because you are actually *under*nourished—right here, in the United States!

Are You Really Hungry, or Are Your Toxic Cells Just Trying to Unload Their Toxic Burden?

Our air is polluted, our water is impure, and our food definitely isn't what it used to be. On top of that, there is an endless supply of drugs: over-the-counter, under-the-counter, recreational, and those your doctor prescribes. In addition, we have eliminated most of the natural ways to remove toxins: A reduced number of saunas, no sweat lodges, less movement, less sweating in the summer because of air conditioners, and less sweating from physical labor have all led to an increase in toxic buildup.

You can reclaim your health by going on a 1-day-fasting cleanse, shutting off the air conditioner once in a while, and drinking herbal teas that promote gentle purification. But the most important part is that you provide healthy food for yourself and your family. In Chapter 7, you will learn how an anti-inflammatory diet can reduce your toxic burden and reset your metabolism.

Are You Really Hungry, or Does Your Parasympathetic Overdrive Make You Eat More?

Your body has two modes of operation: sympathetic and parasympathetic. Together, these are called the autonomic nerve system. The autonomic nerve system regulates involuntary actions such as blushing, sweating, sexual arousal, heart rate, bowel peristalsis (the forward movement of feces through the intestine), and swallowing. All of these functions are governed by a very ancient part of your brain that sits at the place where your brain goes into your spinal cord.

The *sympathetic* branch of the autonomic nerve system governs the *fight-or-flight* reflexes. If needed, the autonomic nerve system increases oxygen intake in your lungs, lets your heart beat faster, brings more blood to your deep muscles, and dilates your pupils—all of which you need to fight an enemy or to run away.

The *parasympathetic* branch concerns itself with your *rest-and-digest* functions, also called *feed-and-breed*. If you are constantly eating and drinking, day and night, and barely moving, your body is only concerned with digestion. When your parasympathetic drive is switched on, you store sugar in your liver; when it is switched off, you use all the stored sugar and fat.

Parasympathetic overdrive leads to weight gain.[37] But we can turn from parasympathetic drive to sympathetic drive by taking up a little bit of exercise, going for a short daily walk, using the stairs instead of the elevator, moving around the room a bit as we work or talk on the phone, or even stretching. In short, you can make the *fight-or-flight* reflexes work for you by incorporating small amounts of movement throughout every day.

Are You Really Hungry, or Are Your Olfactory Nerves Making Food Ever More Appealing to You?

Food just smells too darn good to you. You can't walk by a bakery without going in and buying a brown bag full of muffins, fresh breads, croissants, bagels, tarts, and cookies. But what spurs this impulse?

Olfactory nerves—the cells responsible for smelling—are situated close to your limbic system, which is responsible for your feelings. Aromatherapy, for instance, uses the close relationship between smell and emotions.[38] Some people are more prone to follow their noses than others are, and everybody falls easier for a smell when they are hungry than when they are full.[39] But to be safe, whenever something smells appetizing, ask yourself if you are truly hungry. Often, you'll find that you're not.

Are You Really Hungry, or Are Your Estrogen and Progesterone Levels Unbalanced?

Estrogen and progesterone are two hormones that have to be in fine balance in the female body. It is well known that with estrogen excess, the body layers on more fat and women gain weight. Estrogen sends hunger signals to your brain, an effect that is independent of leptin.[40] Nevertheless, unbalanced estrogen levels can lead to insulin resistance and type 2 diabetes. Of course, genetics determine how much estrogen relative to progesterone a woman has in her body. But modern life may add to a woman's natural estrogen levels. And certain estrogen sources are unwanted—and often unrecognized. These include:

- Hormone replacement therapy (HRT) during menopause.

- Soybeans, which provide phytoestrogens. Occasionally, those phyto-estrogens are a good thing, but soy has been marketed as a wonder food and, therefore, is found in many processed foods. Plus, nonorganic soy is gentically manipulated, and the jury is still out on whether or not this might be harmful. Since genetically modified organisms (GMOs) do not need to be labeled in the United States, you can only be sure to avoid them by buying organic soy.

- Dairy products, which increase estrogens and decrease anti-estrogens— a double hazard to put on fat and gain weight.[41] They also increase your risk of developing breast and endometrial cancer.[42]

Are You Really Hungry, **or Are You Overexercising?**

When you exercise, your leptin level goes up, signaling satiety to your brain. But if you exercise very hard—or overexercise—your leptin level falls and you become hungry again.[43] Sounds simple. But overexercising means different things to different people. It depends on your genes, how your body is built, and your exercise history. If you are overweight and the farthest you've walked has been from your bed to your car or from your sofa to your bed, a short walk will do wonders for you. If you have been a competitive athlete since your teens, you will need more for a perfect balance. Either way, it's important to know: There is such a thing as exercising too much.

SIGNS OF OVEREXERCISING

- Thinking about exercise and your body too much (several times a day)
- Annoying your friends by talking about nothing else but exercise (which has to be carefully distinguished from genuine, fruitful enthusiasm)
- Feeling upset or irritable if you have to skip your exercise for a day
- Putting your exercise ahead of everything else: family, friends, work
- Experiencing frequent injuries: An injury is often a sign that your body is overtaxed.

If you recognize any of these signs, it does not mean you should stop altogether, only that you should reevaluate your goals and means. Are you overtraining? Are you pushing yourself too hard? Is your present level of exercise maintainable?

Are You Really Hungry, **or Are Your Chemically Damaged Mitochondria Piling On the Fat?**

If you look at a map of regions with high obesity rates in the United States, you may be surprised to find that it looks alarmingly similar to a map that shows where the mitochondria-damaging herbicide atrazine is used most. While that is not proof of cause, science has provided some good arguments supporting why atrazine may indeed add to the burden of obesity in our country.

Chronic exposure to atrazine in the drinking water—which is exactly the scenario in our predominantly agrarian states—hurts our mitochondria and leads to insulin resistance and obesity.[44] We've already discussed how obesity itself damages mitochondria by putting so much fat into the cells that the poor cells have no breathing room for proper function. But herbicides also lead to decreased mitochondrial function. This, in turn, piles up fat and increases your appetite, which hampers those little cell batteries even further. Needless to say, atrazine might only be the tip of the iceberg. There are innumerable artificial molecules out there that could damage your delicate cell mechanisms.

To fight this chemical damage, try to filter your water and eat fresh vegetables every day. Both of these measures help your mitochondria unload their toxins.

Are You Really Hungry, or Does Your Low-Fat Diet Leave You Empty?

One medical myth I stopped believing long ago: Fats are bad for us. Even when I felt I was giving the best medical advice to my patients by telling them to "cut down on the fat," I was never really able to cut out fats myself. I grew so incredibly hungry without them! So I have slowly come to the conclusion that I probably gave bad advice to my patients. What I advise now is to incorporate good fats into every meal: Use olive oil for salads, coconut oil for frying, ghee (clarified butter) when a buttery taste is desirable, and occasionally a bit of European-style cultured butter (very occasionally!).

For the longest time we have been told that eating fat makes us fat and sick. Now it turns out that most fats are not contributing to obesity, but that sugars and starches are the main culprits![45] At one point, when heart disease skyrocketed in the mid-20th century, scientists came to the conclusion that fats were not only making us sick. But in the last 10 years, their thinking has become more refined, and now we know that not all fats are bad. Certain fats are good for us, and even some saturated fats like coconut oil and ghee[46] can be beneficial to our health! But avoid bad fats, which include everything fried and most salad dressings, except those made from scratch with olive oil. Also avoid highly overprocessed or overheated fats and trans fats like hydrogenated oils, margarine, shortening, deep-frying fats, and hardened coconut oil (invented for a longer shelf life).

You should also avoid animal fat, unless it's organic meat that comes from livestock that has been grass-fed and kept outside during its lifetime. Presently, our food animals are stuffed with unnatural foods (corn!), doused with antibiotics and other modern medicines, kept in narrow pens without sunlight, and restricted from movement. When we eat their unhealthy flesh, we are getting sick, too.[47]

Because fats were looked down upon for such a long time, low-fat diets were popular and considered "heart healthy"—remember? But a low-fat diet deprives you of very essential nutrients. For instance, all of the fat-soluble vitamins (A, D, E, and K) cannot be absorbed without fat present. A diet low in fat is, by definition, either high in carbohydrates or in proteins.[48] High in carbohydrates often means simple carbohydrates—sugars and starches, and especially high-fructose corn syrup—which are clearly producing obesity and diabetes. A diet high in proteins can easily overload your kidneys and can lead to gout.[49]

As bad as this may sound, it gets worse: A diet low in fat can leave you rather hungry. Of the three basic food groups—carbs, fats, and proteins—fats lead to satiety fastest and reduce the amount of food you consume.[50]

Are You Really Hungry, or Does Your Bread-and-Cereal Habit Leave You Insatiable, Irritable, and Thick in the Middle?

Grains have been overrated ever since agriculture began 5,000 to 10,000 years ago. And no wonder, either: They play right into your endorphin system, leaving you feeling good—and bloated, fat, inflamed, and diabetic.

Grains taste too good, especially in combination with fat and sugar, and they push our pleasure buttons. We will never get away from them until we view them with a bit more suspicion. Sure, at a certain point in history grains helped to prevent starvation. Many more children survived to adulthood after agriculture was invented and with it, bread and milk. But now, the drawbacks of grains have become clearer.

1. Starvation is less of a problem now in the United States. Instead, we have an obesity problem, and grains deliver simple carbohydrates—namely sugars and starches—which are at the root of obesity.

2. Grains contain antinutrients like lectins—especially in the hull and bran parts—because grains are seeds, and plants want their precious seeds to grow into new plants, not to be eaten. Lectins are designed to

hurt the one who eats the seeds. So these antinutrients harm our intestines and, therefore, increase inflammation in our bodies, further contributing to diabetes. Diabetics should, consequently, eat even whole grains sparingly and instead try to get most of their complex carbohydrates from vegetables.

3. Grains are addictive, and having to go without them makes people cranky and irritable. If you build your meal around vegetables with a bit of protein and fat, and you incorporate only small amounts of grains, you will be satisfied. Simple carbohydrates like bread, pancakes, doughnuts, spaghetti, macaroni, sub rolls, lasagna, toast, cookies, cakes, and muffins are all "s'more" foods: One can never get enough.

Are You Really Hungry, or Does Your High-Dairy Diet Intensify Your Appetite?

If I wanted to get people to eat more vegetables, the easiest thing to do would be to smother those veggies in cheese and cream. After all, anything tastes great covered with cheese because it has a taste we can't resist. It is a taste that offers calories, which were vitally important throughout most of history, when food was scarce. But food is no longer scarce in the United States, and consuming dairy only offers extra, unneeded calories and bodily destruction.

So how do milk and dairy products damage our bodies? It's not because they contain fat (butterfat), but because the milk proteins inflame our guts.[51] In my opinion, dairy is, together with sugar, the most inflammatory food in the standard American diet (SAD). And you may be interested to know that a study performed on over 4,000 British women ages 60–79 found that subjects who reported never consuming milk had a 20 percent reduced chance of developing insulin resistance than those who drank either whole milk or low-fat milk.[52] Unfortunately, however, the inflammation that leads to obesity and diabetes is only part of the problem with dairy.

Dairy tastes good, so we eat more of it than we should. But it also makes us sick. For adults, it is an unnatural, slow-poison food that is linked to pimples, obesity, heart disease, dementia, allergies, asthma, cancer, depression, arthritis, autoimmune disease, and a host of other disorders.[53–65] Why is milk linked to so many diseases? It is highly inflammatory, damaging virtually every organ in your body.[66–68] The proteins found in milk (and all milk products) are at the root of inflammation. We have been told for a long time that butterfat is bad for us, which is why you find long rows of skim milk, low-fat milk, and all the other low-fat dairy products like yogurt and cheese in your supermarket. In low-fat products you get less fat, and consequently more protein—exactly the substance that promotes inflammation in your body.

It turns out that some of the fat in milk might actually be good for us (in moderation). On the other hand, phytanic fatty acid, another fat found in dairy and beef (and probably the culprit if you have an allergic reaction to both), has been shown to induce cancer.[69] If you have asthma, drinking milk exacerbates it, not because you have a genuine milk allergy, but because your poor chronically inflamed body lowers the threshold at which it reacts to any allergen.

As you can see, consuming dairy in any form is linked to numerous health problems, most notably inflammation. Simply cutting dairy from your diet will go a long way toward reducing your inflammation-caused diabetes and your constant hunger. See Chapter 7 for inflammation-reducing dairy substitutions.

Are You Really Hungry, or Do Artificial Sweeteners Make You Want to Keep Eating?

If you use artificial sweeteners, you will never lose your sweet tooth and will always crave sugary foods.[70] And sugar will fuel inflammation and spike your insulin levels, leading you down the path to diabetes. Many sugar substitutes are much sweeter than sucrose (table sugar), which will only make it harder to lose your sugar habit. Worse, artificial sweeteners have been linked to numerous health concerns: neurotoxicity, gastrointestinal problems, cancers, headaches, kidney disease, palpitations, and anxiety.[71-79]

Artificial sweeteners have also been linked to weight gain, even beyond the calorie input. What this means is that, in some weird way, sugar substitutes affect the mechanisms by which your body regulates sugar intake and metabolism. No, sweeteners are not sugar—but they may trigger insulin and decrease leptin even faster than sugar! And they fool your brain into thinking that you didn't eat anything, which causes you to keep reaching for something else to eat.

If you find that you want to eat something sweet, reach for ripe fruit. Once your inflammation and diabetes are under control, you can occasionally indulge in dried fruit, like raisins and apples. And rarely, you can also allow honey and maple syrup in a dish. Stevia is another sweet treat you may include in your diet because it's not an artificial sweetener: It comes from a plant and actually has anti-inflammatory properties.[80]

Are You Really Hungry, or Are Tasty AGE Particles Making You Load Your Plate?

High-heat processing of nearly any food can create toxins called advanced glycation end products (AGEs). AGEs are aptly named because they accelerate aging by producing inflammation in your body, creating a metabolic environment that favors diabetes.[81] And because AGE products mostly taste so good—think grilled foods—you tend to eat more than your share. By encouraging you to eat more, AGEs further our obesity epidemic.

Not only does high heat turn good foods into unhealthy fare, but drying, frying, smoking, grilling, and pasteurization can, too. Suddenly, warnings against eating processed foods appear in a new light: It is not only *what* goes into processed foods that can hurt you, but also *how* the foods are processed, which can cause even more damage. A study that lowered the intake of AGE particles without changing the participants' diets led, in a short time, to lower inflammation markers.[82]

Once you ingest AGE particles, they cling to your cells, oxidizing them. And if you know that antioxidants are good for you, you can imagine that oxidizing is harmful. High oxidant levels create oxidative stress and damage your cells, promoting inflammation and a diabetic state.

Are You Really Hungry, or Has Your Body Been Invaded by a Fattening Germ?

Intriguing new science shows that past infection with adenovirus 36 sets people up for higher body mass.[83] Earlier experiments with mice, rats, and primates had suggested this might be the case, but this new study links obesity and viral infection in a human population. Even more titillating is the fact that several other infections are linked to human obesity, insulin resistance, and/or metabolic syndrome: CDV (Canine distemper virus), RAV-7 (Rous-associated virus-7), BDV (Borna disease virus), Scrapie agent (a prion), adenovirus 36, avian adenovirus SMAM-1, *Helicobacter pylori*, *Chlamydia pneumonia*, *Porphyromonas gingivalis*, HCV (hepatitis C virus), and HIV (human immunodeficiency virus). And the mechanism by which the germs make you gain weight? Inflammation.[84] So what does all of this mean? Choosing an anti-inflammatory lifestyle becomes even more important.

Moving Forward

By now you should be able to identify with at least a few of the hunger culprits listed in this chapter. Not all of the culprits carry the same weight, and not all of them apply to your personal situation. But the sum of these points gives you an idea of how things were stacked against you and possibly even led to your diabetes diagnosis.

Keep in mind that feeling hungry is good: It keeps you on your toes. Feeling hungry is where healing starts, but it is not where it needs to end. You can reeducate your mind and your gut. Your body can learn to crave better foods. Your mind can learn that there is more to life than instant gratification through your mouth.

Identifying your triggers is half the battle. So now you need to ask yourself: What can I do to change my future? To reverse your diabetes, you must first reduce the inflammation that caused it. And the only way to do this is to change your life. If you find all of the advice confusing, think about where we humans came from, and recreate in your daily life as many of those ancient moments as you can: Eat more vegetables, go outside more often, sleep enough hours, shut off all the distracting machines every once in a while, move a little bit. After all, your old habits got you into this trouble, and now that you're armed with the knowledge of what makes you exhausted and voracious, you can begin to change your ways—and change your life.

PART 3

Curing Your Diabetes

6

The Five Health Essentials

for a Diabetes-Free Life

In order to change,
we must be sick and tired
of being sick and tired.

—AUTHOR UNKNOWN

How we choose to live can make us sick. But how we choose to live can also heal us. Eating more nutritious food, having less stress, and incorporating small amounts of movement can—and will—reduce the chronic inflammation in your body. But don't expect a quick fix. Instead, you will begin by rethinking what your body and soul need because diabetes is not just an inconvenience preventing you from eating all the cake you want. It is a very serious condition that requires serious reconsideration of your lifestyle.

You already know what does not work:

- **Calorie restriction.** You gained weight because, try as you might, you can't prevent yourself from overeating. For example, let's say your body requires an intake of 2,500 calories each day, but you overate for several days or weeks in a row. As a result, you suddenly restrict your caloric allowance to 1,200 calories in the hope of getting yourself back on track. Why would it suddenly work? Willpower may push you for a while, but it will be almost impossible to stick with this program until you reach your goal weight.

  What happens is this: You restrict yourself for a while, but then comes the ravenous hunger. When this hunger hits, you binge and fall off the wagon. Consequently, you feel defeated, forget about your diet, and buy your clothes a size larger. Then, when a new diet appears on the market, you fall for it again and repeat the cycle.

  The emphasis is always on which diet will "melt away the pounds": the all-eggs diet, the low-carb diet, the all-carbs diet, the vegan diet, the vegetarian diet, the macrobiotic diet, the mailed-to-your-home diet, and more. None of these diets work for long, and their downfall is always the same: You're simply not getting what your body needs.

- **Quick weight reduction.** Again, severe calorie restriction and an enormous amount of willpower will only get you so far. In the long run, they will always fail because nature will see to it that you don't starve. You will feel like a failure, but the fault lies with the wrong approach and the wrong foods chosen, not with you.

- **Appetite suppressants.** Some work, although with severe adverse effects. The amphetamine-like substances are known for heart problems and mania[1-2] and, therefore, come with restrictions and warnings. Phentermine, which is in the same family, targets the hormones in your brain and puts extra stress on both your body and your mind. It also causes high blood pressure, increased heart rate, and sleeplessness. Yes, you may lose weight, but only because you're putting extra stress on your mind and your body, which makes you age faster.[3] Ephedrine, an herb in the same pharmacological group as phentermine, has been banned for over-the-counter use because of those dangers.[4]

- **Excessive exercise.** Exercising too much makes you hungry, exacerbating your problem. On the other hand, moderate exercise actually suppresses appetite.[5]

- **The combination of reduced calories and exercise.** Just recently (the scientific paper has not yet been published), the Joslin Diabetes Center in Boston prematurely canceled an 11-year study on the effects of a reduced-calorie diet and exercise regimen. Why? There was no evidence that the incorporation of such a diet and exercise plan reduced mortality. Continuing the study was, therefore, deemed unethical.[6]

  You may have read the pessimistic reports in newspapers and magazines. The study seemed to be well designed: More than 5,000 overweight to obese people with type 2 diabetes were put on a low-calorie diet and a regimen of "moderate" exercise for nearly 3 hours per week. It's hard to determine what "moderate" signifies here: In my experience with typical patients, 3 hours per week in the gym is, statistically, not "moderate." Those who exercise at least 3 hours a week are accustomed to making fitness a part of their daily lives, but most people with diabetes feel that they don't have enough energy to maintain such a time-consuming fitness schedule. But we know what "low-calorie diet" means: severely reduced portions of the same standard American diet (SAD) that brought those people into their diabetic states in the first place. There was no consideration of the real nutritional needs of people diagnosed with type 2 diabetes.

  By the way, there was a good outcome: Although the people in the study group did not seem much healthier when the study was canceled, they did use less medication. And on average, they lost 5 percent of their body weight. As a result, it's clear to me that while the exercise portion of the study seemed to have worked, the *diet* did not—and now we know why.

If none of the above methods work to cure your diabetes or achieve lasting weight loss, it stands to reason that a new approach is needed—one that works with your natural survival instincts, not against them. As a Natural Medicine physician (who is also trained in conventional medicine), I want to encourage you to listen to your body, because only *you* can feel what's going on inside.

The Principles of Natural Medicine

A conventional doctor is not trained to encourage you to take care of yourself. This physician is so eager to take care of you that sometimes it does not even occur to her that she has to consult with you in the matter of your health. After all, *she* attended medical school, and *she* knows everything about the human body. But not every human body is the same—a fact that most conventional physicians overlook. Fortunately, Natural Medicine physicians are aware of this and, therefore, practice according to the six Principles of Natural Medicine[7] listed below.

1. **First, do no harm.** Utilize the most natural, least invasive, and least toxic therapies. "Do no harm" was introduced by the famous Greek physician Hippocrates (c. 460 BC–c. 370 BC); it was contained in an oath all young doctors had to pledge before being allowed to practice medicine. These days, most medical schools have dropped the Hippocratic Oath. Natural Medicine still adheres to the principle that the cure should not be more damaging than the disease and, therefore, uses milder herbs and natural methods.

2. **The healing power of nature.** Acute diseases such as severe infections and trauma certainly need acute conventional medical care. But chronic conditions often stem from bad lifestyle choices and are reversible, to a degree: If you take away what damages your body and replace it with better habits, your body has a chance to heal itself.

3. **Identify and treat the causes.** It is not good enough to simply give a diagnosis and provide a pill if the condition originates from living against the natural grain. Look beyond the symptoms to the underlying cause.

4. **Doctor as teacher.** Literally, *doctor* means *teacher*. The physician does not merely assign prescriptions, procedures, and surgeries to the patient. It's more important to educate patients in the steps to achieving and maintaining health.

5. **Treat the whole person.** The physician has to view the body as an integrated whole in all its physical and spiritual dimensions, taking into account that bodies and lives are different and that one size does not fit all. The physician is dependent upon the patient's input, his observations, his beliefs, and his desires. The physician has to respect that the patient *owns his own health*.

6. **Prevention.** In old China, a physician was paid as long as everyone remained healthy. If someone in the family fell ill, the payment stopped, as the physician had not done his job correctly. This practice no longer exists; but at the very least, physicians should focus on overall health, wellness, and disease prevention.

Natural Medicine versus Conventional Medicine

There are numerous differences between Natural Medicine and conventional medicine, but the one common thread is that both should be evidence-based, whenever possible. Both kinds of medicine are still evolving and should be practiced together for a more comprehensive approach. While conventional medicine is the best approach for acute diseases and issues such as trauma, heart attacks, or strokes, Natural Medicine is the better option when addressing prevention, chronic disease, or rehabilitation.[8]

Natural	Conventional
Patient-centered	Diagnosis-centered
Stages-oriented	Diagnosis-oriented
Individualized dosages	Standardized dosages
Natural herbs	Synthetic drugs
Underresearched	Heavily researched
Synergy of herbal compounds	Isolated chemicals
Traditional wisdom	Efficiency-driven
Disease as imbalance	Disease as enemy
Mind-body medicine	Mind and body addressed in different medical specialties
Holistic	Specialized
Recovery-oriented	Number-oriented
Inexpensive	Expensive
Best for chronic disease	Best for acute disease
Early prevention	Late intervention
Slow improvement	Rapid improvement
Few side effects	Many side effects
Compassionate	Analytical

Adapted from Sato Y (ed.), *Introduction to Kampo: Japanese Traditional Medicine* (Tokyo: Elsevier Japan, 2005).

Listening to Your Body

A stalk of Brussels sprouts once survived in my fridge while I was traveling to the West Coast. Upon my return, I suddenly had the vision that I would like to eat those green little roses for breakfast—and with raisins, of all things!

I knew I would have to wake up a bit earlier that morning to actually cook the strange breakfast. But by this point in my life, I took my gut feelings seriously. So I woke up early and cooked my breakfast of Brussels sprouts and raisins. And it was delicious.

So why do I take my hunches seriously? Well, I figure my body is trying to fill a slight deficiency. But then again, I don't follow hunches for marshmallows or M&M's, because they are unnatural (although I have turned to dark chocolate if I had a craving for something sweet).

Here's another example: Thirty years ago, I woke up one Sunday with an urge to visit a specific museum, which was hundreds of miles away. And somehow I made it there within the following month. Ultimately, through that museum (it's a long, convoluted story), I met my future husband!

You may be wondering why I'm discussing something as unscientific as hunches. The answer is because we are bombarded by health news, scientific breakthroughs, and advertisements for new superfoods every day, and it is hard to find our way through this maze of information. Early on, I decided that I needed to see—and feel—the difference in my body, my mood, and even my soul before I believed any new health hype. And it has never led me wrong.

For instance, I always craved more fat in my diet than medical wisdom allowed me to eat. My brain did not function well without enough good fat, mostly olive oil. At that time, I was still timid and told my patients to stick to the official line in conventional medicine—namely, to cut out fat. But at home, I bathed my vegetables in all the fat I desired. Interestingly, my weight remained stable, contrary to what medicine was teaching at that time.

So now, when you take a new supplement, think about the reason behind your decision. Do you take it because your doctor/your herbalist/your acupuncturist/your friend/your newspaper/a Web site told you to do so? Or do you take it because it makes you feel so much better than before—because you're listening to your body's needs?

Everybody tells you what is "good for you": advertisers, vendors, physicians, and even your family and friends. They all clamor for your attention by trying to sell you their versions of "health." But how do you make up your own mind about what is healthy? Should you believe every published research study—some good, some bad—or the myriad of business interests that want your money? And will that new fad diet recommended by your friends improve your health and cure your diabetes? In short, the answer is no.

After nearly 40 years of studying health, I believe the only way to achieve true health is to use your body as nature intended. And by doing this, you will never go hungry, never restrict calories, and never have to join a gym. Instead, you will enjoy a delicious, filling meal plan while incorporating small amounts of exercise here and there that can easily be slipped into your day. But diet and exercise alone won't cure you. Health rests on a larger foundation than this. To eliminate the inflammation in your body and ultimately cure your diabetes, you must incorporate The Five Health Essentials.

The Five Health Essentials

Sebastian Kneipp (1821–1897) was the first person to develop a Natural Medicine treatment system. Interestingly, he was not a physician, but a Catholic priest. While in seminary, he fell ill with tuberculosis, as so many people did in the 19th century. Desperate for a solution, Kneipp found literature claiming that cold water therapy could cure tuberculosis and subsequently jumped into the Danube River during the middle of winter. Following many short cold dunks in the river, he cured his tuberculosis and developed a water cure that helped many.

After Kneipp was banned to a remote nunnery for his "water splashing," he began to self-experiment with herbs and other measures his herbalist mother had taught him. As a result, he expanded his system of healing to include food, herbs, movement, and balance. Together with water, these elements became known as The Five Health Essentials of Natural Medicine. And thanks to modern science, we now know that each of these five components fights the dangerous inflammation in our bodies.

1. **Food.** Your eating habits have led to the chronic inflammation that caused your diabetes. But research has shown that eating anti-inflammatory foods (fresh vegetables, good proteins, and healthy fats packed with anti-diabetic phytochemicals) will eliminate the inflammation in your body.[9] In fact, a 2004 study in the *Journal of Nutrition* showed that a greater frequency of consumption of fruits and vegetables was associated with lower C-reactive protein and homocysteine concentrations in elderly men. Interestingly, with each additional serving of fruit and vegetable

intake, the risk of having high c-reactive protein and homocysteine concentrations decreased by 21 percent and 17 percent, respectively.[10] So you'll leave behind factory-processed "food" filled with sugar, starches, bad fats, and inferior proteins, and (re)discover how a meal can be tasty and wholesome. And because your new diet will consist of delicious, filling food, you'll never miss the inflammatory junk food you used to crave.

2. **Herbs.** You will include herbs (otherwise known as Nature's apothecary) in your teas, add them to your food for spice and flavor, and use them as medicine for minor ailments such as an oncoming cold or an upset stomach. By focusing on herbs with anti-inflammatory and anti-diabetic properties, you'll lower your blood sugar levels while fighting inflammation.[11]

3. **Movement.** Don't sign up for that gym just yet! I have some proven recommendations for little *1-minute exercises* that will make all the difference in how you feel and how your diabetes will recede.

4. **Balance.** A healthy, diabetes-free life is not achieved simply by incorporating a new diet and a little exercise. It comes from an all-around balanced life, including refreshing sleep, rewarding relationships, music, art, the great outdoors, and a spiritual interest. Sleep deprivation furthers inflammation and diabetes, while fulfilling pastimes and relationships have been shown to lower stress-related parameters such as blood pressure, lipids, immune function, and inflammation markers.

5. **Water.** The rule of thumb here is to fight inflammation by using *cold* water on the outside and *warm* water on the inside. And a study in the *European Journal of Applied Physiology* has shown that exposure to cold water at least three times a week can aid in weight loss by increasing metabolic rate due to shivering.[12] In addition, a 2012 study published in the *Journal of Clinical Investigation* revealed that subjects who were kept cold (not the point of shivering) for 3 hours experienced an 80 percent increase in their metabolic rates.[13] Don't worry: Occasionally, a warm bath is acceptable. But your beverages should always be at room temperature or warmer, and they should be as natural as possible.

In the following chapters, you will learn more about how The Five Health Essentials target the inflammation in your body and will help you to reclaim your health and your diabetes-free life. So let's get started!

Food

The doctor of the future will no longer
treat the human frame with drugs,
but rather will cure and prevent disease
with nutrition.

—THOMAS EDISON (1847–1931)

You Are What You Eat

There are two truths you can't get around when it comes to food.

1. Cause and effect reign over the laws of Nature and apply to you, too. So
   if you eat pizza, doughnuts, and ice cream, you will get a pizza–
   doughnuts–ice cream body.

2. We are living in modern times, but your body has ancient biochemistry
   and ancient physiology and, therefore, requires certain things in order
   to function well. If you deprive your body of what it requires, you will
   become sick.

From these two truths, we can envision the types of meals that nurture
your ancient physiology.

- **Your meals should be healthy—heart-healthy, brain-healthy, etc.** So how do we classify foods as healthy or unhealthy? Simply stated: Healthy foods fight inflammation. This translates mostly into vegetables, vegetables, and more vegetables—though not exclusively. Each meal should be planned around two or three vegetables (two aboveground and one underground, or root), one grain or legume, and one protein. Meat, fish, and eggs should be an afterthought and don't need to be served every day.

- **Your meals should be similar to the foods our ancestors ate when they were living in caves.** But don't assume that we could ever eat exactly as they ate because those foods do not exist anymore. And even if they did, they would most likely not appeal to you: carrots the size of your pinkie, leathery green leaves, wild meats with barely a gram of fat, crab apples, and grubs. Their food was also bitter. Therefore, bitter foods are also beneficial for us.

- **Your meals should be made up of organic, local, and in-season items whenever possible because the process of organic *farming* puts more healthy molecules into the plant you're eating.**[1] If your food is *local* that means it retains more of those healthy molecules during transportation than food that's shipped from far away. And by eating food that's *in season*, you'll avoid having the same plants in your system too often, thus reducing your risk of developing a food allergy.

- **Your meals should be customized.** Coming from different continents, climates, landscapes, and races, human beings have different genetic backgrounds and, therefore, have different food requirements and food preferences; *your* diet has to nourish and satisfy *your* body, not mine. So while I will provide you with the relative quantities of fats, proteins, and carbohydrates you should consume, specific quantities do vary from person to person based on your genetic background, physical activity level, and climate. This point, however, does not mean that it's permissible to eat doughnuts instead of broccoli, for example, just because that's what you're craving. If you want to cure your diabetes, you have to learn to prefer broccoli to that sugary, starchy doughnut.

  A study showed that infants need to be exposed to a new food repeatedly before they start to seek it out.[2] And adults, with their less impressionable brains, need even more time. So try those mustard greens at least a dozen times before you label them inedible.

- **Your meals should promote weight loss.** Nature's laws are at work here, too: If you need to lose weight, you have to restrict calories until you reach your ideal weight. But who wants to spend time counting calories? By eating foods that fight inflammation, you don't have to count calories. Instead, you just have to add fats and proteins to your meals in order to be satisfied—and to remain satisfied for a longer time. And keep this in mind: You can only keep portions smaller if you eat high-quality food, not empty calories. So focus on eating quality, filling foods, and remember to avoid using artificial sweeteners, which fool your body into thinking that you have not eaten at all and ultimately cause you to eat more.

- **Your meals should be flexible.** Our forefathers, the hunter-gatherers, never could aspire to balanced meals; they simply ate what they found or hunted, and over time it evened out. If you live alone and don't want to cook larger, more diverse meals every day, try the Tibetan Alternative, where you only eat a single item at each meal, rotating from a vegetable to a piece of meat, beans, fruit, and so on. In the end, you will have a balanced week of meals.

- **Your meals should not be planned around your medications**—instead, your medications should be planned around your meals. This is a hint for people on the blood thinner warfarin (Coumadin): All greens contain vitamin K, which counteracts warfarin (Coumadin). But you should not avoid greens—just make sure to eat them in roughly equal amounts every day. Physicians often tell their Coumadin patients to not eat greens. I'm telling you to eat greens regularly and talk to your doctor about adjusting your medication accordingly—not the other way around.

In short, do not believe that there is a "magic bullet" diet—one that lets you lose weight effortlessly "while eating all your favorite foods"! This kind of thinking and advertisement are what led to your diagnosis in the first place. Your favorite foods are likely highly inflammatory, and research has shown that inflammatory foods promote weight gain and diabetes.[3] So in order to truly cure your diabetes, you have to change your life—beginning with your diet.

A SAD Story

You interact with the world primarily through your digestive tract because food particles are absorbed into your bloodstream during digestion. With contact this intimate, the chance of harming your body increases—especially if the food you eat is furthering inflammation. Of course there are safety checks, like when you feel disgust at a bad smell, instinctively spit out nasty-tasting substances that might be poisonous, or vomit and experience diarrhea to purge rotten foods and viruses. But these safety checks deal with *acutely* harmful matter, not with chronically injuring inflammation that accumulates over the years. Chronic harm sneaks in unnoticed and comes from two sides.

- Foods **devoid** of the many chemical compounds that plants provide and which our cells need to maintain, repair, and rebuild our bodies.
- Foods **loaded** with modern factory-made molecules that your body can't recognize as harmful and which, therefore, pass by unchecked.

When you combine both of these types of toxic food, as happens with the Standard American Diet (SAD), it creates disease. And currently we are exporting our SAD into every known corner of the world. With the SAD, we live in a state of constant intestinal inflammation—and from there the affliction moves to our skin (pimples, psoriasis, eczema), brain (depression, stroke, dementia, Parkinson's), joints (arthritis), heart (heart attack, clogging of arteries), and intestines (leaky gut, colitis). We have seen this firsthand in the mind-blowing epidemic of diabetes and obesity in the United States. And research has shown that both diabetes and obesity are *systemic*, meaning that they affect every single organ in your body.[4]

There is no doubt that the common link is the food we eat: Harmful (pro-inflammatory) food builds weak cells and tissues and produces inflammation inside your body, while good (anti-inflammatory) food builds healthy cells and tissues and quenches inflammation.

In fact, a 2005 study published in the *American Journal of Clinical Nutrition* showed that subjects who consumed an inflammatory diet high in soft drinks, refined grains, and processed meat, but low in wine, coffee, and vegetables were two to three times more likely to develop type 2 diabetes. Furthermore, this dietary pattern was strongly related to inflammatory markers, leading the researchers to believe that this diet may increase chronic inflammation in the body.[5] By eating the good, anti-inflammatory foods, you nourish your cells directly. But these foods also have an indirect positive effect: Research has shown that they foster healthy gut bacteria, which in turn will enhance resistance to infections and colds, increase mineral and vitamin absorption, protect against colon cancer, lower blood pressure, improve cholesterol, and reduce inflammation.[6] So naturally, you don't want to keep eating the harmful foods or meals that caused your troubles in the first place. Instead, you want to plan your meals around the anti-inflammatory foods that will ultimately eliminate your inflammation and diabetes—and you can. All you have to do is learn the difference.

The French Paradox

In the early 1990s, American scientists and the American public firmly believed that fat was the root of all dietary evils, and the low-fat diet craze was at a high point. Then scientists stumbled across a study that showed that French people ate more fat (triple brie and foie gras), drank more wine (a smooth Bordeaux), and smoked more frequently (Gauloises) than their American counterparts, yet they experienced less cardiovascular disease and lived longer.[7] Scientists dubbed this puzzle The French Paradox and began searching for the reason behind this surprising discovery.

As a way of explaining the paradox, scientists came up with these major differences between eating habits in France and the United States.

- The French have their main meal at midday and take more time to enjoy it (2 hours, minimum).
- The French prefer wine over beer. (Wine contains resveratrol, an antioxidant polyphenol that promotes longevity.)[8]
- The French don't snack.
- The French eat more healthy saturated fats, fewer trans fats (fried foods), and fewer hydrogenated fats (margarine and processed food).
- The French eat less sugar, less high-fructose corn syrup (HFCS), and less white starch.

But scientists still couldn't figure it out: Which one was the main culprit? They couldn't decide. While each of these factors plays a role in overall health, the main and often forgotten point is this: The French eat *fresh* food. The *freshness* of food counts, but interestingly, scientists never mentioned freshness, as it did not occur to them. But there is no doubt in my mind that quality food is freshly grown and harvested, not concocted in a lab to tickle your taste buds, manufactured in bulk, and designed for a long shelf life. The French eat fresh. And that, somehow, protects them against other lifestyle mistakes they might make—like smoking.

Do You Need Vitamins or Supplements?

As long as they are in plants or in meats, vitamins are natural substances. What you buy in a bottle, however, is mostly low-quality stuff that's made in a factory—often without much supervision or quality control.

Vitamins from a bottle can't make up for poor food choices. Your vitamins should come from fresh food. Medically speaking, vitamin deficiencies do exist. If your physician diagnoses such a state, by all means take the prescribed pill, but not forever. Your doctor should find out the root cause— why you are deficient in the first place. Often, deficiencies are the result of a poor diet or an inflamed gut that's unable to absorb vitamins.

Having thus warned against vitamin supplements, there are certain vitamins and minerals that often are low in people, and their deficiency can do much harm. Therefore, here are the levels you should ask your physician to check.

- **Vitamin B$_{12}$.** A deficiency leads to anemia, which is reversible if you ingest the vitamin. But it also leads to dementia, and the dementia is irreversible: The cognitive ability will be lost for good. Everybody over the age of 50 should be checked for vitamin B$_{12}$ levels.

- **Vitamin D.** This vitamin has more importance than we ever thought. It was known that vitamin D was important for bone health. But we have learned that a low level is linked to many cancers and other diseases, including multiple sclerosis.[9] For vitamin D (as well as vitamin B$_{12}$), the established "normal" levels might not be enough. Make sure that your levels of vitamin D are at least normal, or even a bit above normal, for your protection.

  Vitamin D is especially important for those with diabetes: A deficiency leads to mild weight gain,[10] which you don't need if you are already

My Food Pyramid Is Topped by Freshness

If the government asked for my opinion on redesigning their food pyramid, one single principle would guide my choices: *freshness*. Freshness would be at

struggling. Vitamin D is manufactured in the layers of your skin under the influence of sunlight. But it can be hard to get the right amount: Light is healthy, but sunburn is not. Inner-city dwellers often do not get enough light, and the darker and older your skin is, the harder it is to get the sunlight through your skin to work on your vitamin D stores.

- **Calcium.** Bones need far more than just calcium: Other minerals, including boron, chromium, manganese, magnesium, phosphorus, potassium, selenium, and sulfur, are also necessary for bone health. Without these other minerals, calcium alone is pretty useless.

  As we discussed, dairy is an unsuitable source of calcium. Your calcium requirements are easily met by making sure your diet includes a variety of vegetables, fruits, legumes, whole grains, and nuts. Actually, the plant world is so abundant in calcium and bone-building minerals that adding vitamin D to milk as a selling argument comes close to being a joke—and a bad one: A 12-year long health study performed on over 77,000 women ages 34 to 59 found that those who consumed the most calcium from milk experienced more fractures than those who rarely drank the substance.[11]

From now on, whenever another article catches your eye, screaming that you need more vitamin A for your eyes, lycopene for your prostate, or resveratrol for longevity, pay close attention. The research is often well done, but science has yet to prove that downing a pill will make you healthier. (And for many vitamins, the opposite is true!) Have your physician check your level of that vitamin, or mineral, or miracle ingredient. Find out which foods contain that exciting new molecule, and eat the whole foods, rather than take the pills.

the top, and freshness would be at the bottom, because there really is no other food than fresh food; everything processed, enriched, manipulated, enhanced, improved, or ready-made is not food, but actually inferior substitutes. These *fake* "foods" do not contain the nutrients needed to build and repair cells, and they ultimately lead to stunted development, depression, dementia, and disease,[12–15] whereas fresh food protects our bodies.

Over the years, scientists have come up with some strange "food" solutions. Don't get me wrong—I think that science has to corroborate everything we do in medicine. But there have been some mistakes in the past, like these.

- **Astronaut food.** In the 1950s, scientists thought they could do away with stinky, "unnecessary" defecation because in space, under conditions of zero gravity, it was a messy business. They developed "astronaut food" that was entirely absorbed into the body, so that nothing had to leave the end of the intestine. Brilliant, right? No—astronauts got sick. Turns out we need the messy, stinky elimination process to get rid of toxins. (That's when the usefulness of fiber in the diet was discovered.)[16]

- **Vitamins.** Scientists thought that vitamins from a bottle were as good as those eaten in foods—until a study found that the vitamin A precursor beta-carotene prevented lung cancer when it was consumed in its natural form, in food, but promoted cancer when it was taken as a supplement.[17] Other studies came to similar conclusions for vitamins A, C, and E. (To learn more about the need for vitamins, see "Do You Need Vitamins or Supplements?" on page 84.)

- **Hydrogenated fats.** In the beginning of the 20th century, industrialization and globalization of food became widespread. A useful fat like coconut oil that came cheap from tropical countries had the one disadvantage that it easily turned rancid during long shipping passages and storage on shelves across the country. Scientists were hailed for their new method of "hydrogenation"—making hard, long-lasting fats from runny, easily spoiling oils. Margarines and shortenings were modern foods, good for every kitchen, and affordable. Unfortunately, the hardening of oils also caused the hardening of arteries and is responsible for the wave of heart disease during the second half of the century.

The list of foods scientists thought they could "improve" on is long, yet it turns out that we are perfectly nourished if we stick to what Nature provides. But what exactly does Nature provide? All plant cells contain small, health-promoting molecules known as *phytonutrients* (*phyto* means *plant*). They repair and maintain your cells and their functions, aid in detoxification, prevent cancers, and—most importantly, for diabetics—reduce inflammation. We are not getting these phytonutrients from our modern foods because everything is milled, refined, homogenized, and purified. As a result of these processes, the plant cells have been destroyed and eliminated. Spaghetti, subs, candy, ice cream, muffins, and doughnuts all have something in common: They are *acellular*, meaning they contain no cells and, hence, no phytonutrients. In fact, when researchers compared ancestral diets with modern acellular foods, they found that our modern foods promote leptin resistance and obesity, which are directly tied to type 2 diabetes.[18] Modern "food" can't nourish you—it only fattens you up. If you eat fresh plant food, you eat whole *cells*, and with them thousands of life-giving, anti-inflammatory compounds.

But wait! What if you don't eat candy and doughnuts, but instead only eat "healthy" processed food? You might think you are doing yourself a favor by eating, for instance, an apple-flavored "nutritional bar"—but think again! That bar has too much sugar, salt, and partially hydrogenated oil, all of which promote obesity, diabetes, and high blood pressure. Why are so-called "diabetic" bars even allowed to have sugar in them?* The bar's oils are hardened to stave off rancidity, but in turn those hydrogenated fats will stiffen your arteries. Its apple flavor is an artificial chemical made in a factory, and it does not contain any of the healthy nutrients found in fresh apples. The bar's ingredients allow it to last forever on store shelves, untouched even by mold. Why would *you* want to eat something that even mold refuses to touch?

While it's true that we cannot eat perfectly healthfully every single time we sit down to dine, we should know what an ideal meal looks like. We know it has to be fresh, which is another way to say it has to contain cells. Cells— live matter—spoil easily. If your food contains cells, it is fresh—unless it is left too long in the fridge or pantry, has been degraded by overcooking or

---

*For instance, a Chocolate Chunk Glucerna Meal Bar for people with diabetes contains 10 grams of sugar and 50 grams of fats. There is no list available telling us where these ingredients came from and what kind of fats there are. This is a chemical concoction of sugar and fat, coming with a non-peer-reviewed study (Fix B, et al., *Diabetes* 52, suppl. 1 (2003): A72) "proving" that this bar is better than other bars for diabetics' health. The truth is, if you pack sugars into enough fats, you slow down their uptake into your bloodstream. But that does not mean that these bars contain anything healthy. One bar of chocolate-flavored unhealthy sugars and fats carries 220 calories.

microwaving, or has been burned excessively during pan-frying, grilling, bar-becuing, or broiling. So let's take a look at how those fresh cells should be filling your plate.

Meals That Heal

You know the three major food groups: carbohydrates, fats, and protein. They feed and fill us and make up the bulk of our meals; they are called *macronutrients*. We used to know that fats were bad, then carbs became bad, and finally too much protein is bad for you, too. You're left wondering if there's anything you *should* eat! This confusion started with science: For the longest time, scientists and doctors thought that those three macronutrients were all we needed. Then, in the early part of the 20th century, they discovered that we would slowly die without vitamins. Well, right now scientists are learning that plants contain many more chemicals essential for our well-being. The three macronutrients prevent starvation, but we really don't suffer much from starvation these days, do we? Macronutrients don't nourish our cells. As it turns out, they *stuff* them. For nourishment, we need micronutrients—those small molecules inside the cells.

Micronutrients provide your body with fuel and energy, but, more importantly, they are the building blocks for your future cells. Foods made up of cells contain nutrients needed to keep your own cells healthy and functioning. What you choose to eat today will determine your health tomorrow. Therefore, you need to eat fresh, mostly vegetal foods (plants). Don't worry—you'll also be eating some carbohydrates, proteins, and good fats (which store energy and aid in important messaging functions in your brain and nerves, and throughout your entire body). But because plants contain more nutrients than fat, protein, and carbs do, they are the most powerful medicine you could take to fight your chronic inflammation.

Anti-Inflammatory Foods versus Pro-Inflammatory Foods

Many things you currently consider to be "foods" are not. Instead, these items are processed, adulterated, refined, diluted, sweetened, salted, or changed in some way. A major challenge faced by people with type 2 diabetes is making the transition back to eating real food. Any "food" with a brand name is not real food anymore because the ingredients have been processed for a long shelf life, which means that most of the beneficial anti-inflammatory components have been lost and salt, sugar, and bad fats and preservatives have been added. See the lists below for an overview of foods that will aid in your fight against diabetes, as well as those that keep inflammation smoldering.

Anti-Inflammatory Foods

- **Fresh vegetables.** All vegetables contain cells and are, therefore, helpful in eliminating the inflammation in your body. But especially helpful are dark leafy greens, which contain bitter substances that can aid in healing diabetes. Root vegetables like rutabaga, parsnip, jicama, red beets, and turnips also have great mineral content and excellent phytonutrients. But they also contain a lot of starches, so while diabetics should eat root vegetables regularly, they should not eat them in great quantities. Aboveground vegetables may be eaten in larger quantities.

  Note: All vegetables are good for you, but members of the nightshade family (tomatoes, potatoes, eggplant, and bell and hot peppers) should be eaten with caution if you already have problems like arthritis, upset stomach, and inflammation. For most of us coming from Europe and Africa, they are late additions to our plates and are harder to assimilate. If they trouble you, leave them out. If they don't trouble you, you can have one nightshade, one time each week.

- **Herbs, fresh and dried.** Herbs will have their own chapter, but they should not be forgotten here as essential foods. They have all the beneficial plant compounds we seek in vegetables—only more so.

- **Legumes (pulses).** These include beans, peas, chickpeas, and lentils, all of which contain healthy fibers and starches that will not spike blood sugar. Legumes contain good proteins, but they are not complete and are typically eaten with rice or corn (or both). But since legumes—like all seeds, grains, and nuts—contain antinutrients, digestion may be difficult. Antinutrients protect plant seeds by acting like little barbs in your intestines, ripping them open and furthering inflammation, but antinutrients (such as lectins) can be destroyed or at least reduced by soaking, cooking, sprouting, and fermentation.

- **Mushrooms.** Fungi have a high protein content and fall between vegetables and meat. They are perfect foods for your immune system and make a good vegetarian meal at least once per week. They are also harder to digest than other vegetables and, therefore, slow down sugar uptake into your bloodstream.

- **Nuts.** These are full of good fats, proteins, and carbs, plus minerals and vitamins—all of which ease inflammation in your body. One could call nuts the perfect food, except that they also contain antinutrients and are more likely than other foods to cause food allergies and digestive problems. To avoid allergies, see "Rotational Schedule for Nuts and Seeds" on page 93.

- **Fresh, local fruit.** Fruit contains soluble and insoluble fiber, natural antioxidants, and vitamins, all of which lower chronic inflammation in your body. But fruit also contains fructose—a dangerous substance for diabetics—so limit yourself to one or two servings a day.

- **Seaweeds.** The vegetables and herbs of the sea can be rather potent, which is why you should eat them on the side, and not as a main dish. But they deliver the goodness of the ocean (salt with many minerals), making them a perfect salt substitute. Their high iodine content prevents a sluggish thyroid from growing a goiter. But too much, especially if your gland is already overfunctioning, can throw you into a thyroid crisis. So if you have hyperthyroidism, avoid them until your condition is under control.

- **Fermented foods.** Foods such as sauerkraut and miso combine the goodness of plants with the value of probiotics (gut-healthy, inflammation-dousing bacteria). Fermenting also reduces antinutrients, making foods less inflammatory and easier to digest. In addition, fermented foods increase saliva, let digestive juices flow, and provide vitamins and minerals that have been "predigested" by bacteria and, therefore, are easily available for the human body—especially vitamin B_{12}.[19] While we humans have lost the ability to manufacture B_{12}, bacteria can still produce it. Sauerkraut was also a traditional source of vitamin C during the winter months, when fresh foods were scarce. Fermented foods are thought to have anti-inflammatory and antibacterial[20-21] effects and to help cleanse a system overloaded with toxins. They reduce fatigue, aging, and definitely diabetes.[22-24]

- **Good fats.** These include organic olive oil, virgin coconut oil, ghee (clarified butterfat), and duck fat, and they all have anti-inflammatory effects. Saturated fats can be healthy when they come from healthy animals; they only turn unhealthy when they come from poorly (and inhumanely) kept livestock.

- **Organic, grass-fed meat.** All of your meat should be from organic, grass-fed, free-roaming animals because this meat is less inflammatory than meat filled with chemicals. And studies have shown that eating red meat does not increase the markers of inflammation in humans.[25]

- **Poultry—organic only.** Contrary to what you have heard, chicken is meat, too, and it's not necessarily better for you than red meat. Your health depends solely on how the cow, chicken, turkey, rabbit, or lamb was raised: Healthy (and health-giving) animals grow outside, under daylight, eating grass and weeds and moving their muscles so that healthy flesh can build up. And the darker the meat, the more iron it provides for your blood cells.

- **Nonfarmed, fresh ocean fish.** Herring, sardines, smelt, shad, anchovies, cod, hake, mackerel, and other ocean fish contain beneficial omega-3 oils. Freshwater fish have less beneficial omega-3 fatty acids than do fish from the ocean. And small fish are less polluted than larger ones.

- **Whole grains.** The grains you eat should be well cooked and served in small portions. (Observe your reaction, though; some people don't tolerate grains because of their antinutritional lectins.)

- **Tea.** This is the perfect beverage to soothe the chronic inflammation in your body—regardless of whether you prefer black, green, or herbal. Drink it without sugar or sugar substitutes. There are so many teas—experiment! In my household, red berry tea and tulsi (holy basil) are favorites. A tea made from garden herbs is nourishing and delicious, but you need an adventurous spirit and plant knowledge.

- **Weeds.** Gather these from your garden or a clean field. Learn how to cook field greens like dandelion and stinging nettle. Take a local herb walk with a guide. And don't harvest and eat any weed that you are not 100 percent sure is safe to consume.

Pro-Inflammatory Foods

- **Dairy.** Milk is designed by Nature to make calves gain weight quickly. And since we are not calves—or even babies any longer—our bodies do not require milk. Contrary to popular belief and advertisement, bone strength does not come from consuming milk and other dairy products, but from plant foods. In fact, dairy is a highly inflammatory food for most people. And more processing ("skimming") does not make it any healthier, only more inflammatory.

- **Sugar.** The sugar industry tries to sell us on the fact that sugar is "natural" because it came from sugarcane. But it's not natural because all the cells within the sugarcane have been eliminated during the refining process. Molasses, at least, retains some of its original minerals, such as iron. Unfortunately, artificial sweeteners have their drawbacks, too—they are suspected to cause many diseases, not to mention weight gain.[26]

- **Refined grains.** These should be avoided altogether, along with milled, fortified, and sweetened grains. Limit your intake of pasta to once a week and avoid refined grains in white bread, cereal, and pizza. To get your diabetes under control, don't eat white starches.

- **Grain-fed meat.** Grain-fed animals that are kept in CAFOs (Concentrated Animal Feeding Operations) are sick and unhealthy because they are not doing what comes naturally to them: grazing, and living outdoors. They are barely kept alive by antibiotics, hormones, and other drugs. When we eat their meat, we become sick, too. And on top of it, processed meats are laced with preservatives, colorings, and artificial flavorings.

- **Tropical fruits.** Because it typically has a higher fructose content than other fruits, people with diabetes should limit their intake of fruits like bananas, oranges, mangoes, papayas, and pineapples to once a week. Also, if your ancestors did not come from hot climates, tropical fruits might be hard for you to digest. Many people eat bananas because their doctors told them that bananas are high in potassium. This is true—but it is also true for many other fruits and vegetables.

- **Bad fats.** Vegetable oils (like corn, soy, and canola), all hydrogenated (or partially hydrogenated) oils, and all oils that have been heated for frying or deep-frying should be avoided.

Rotational Schedule for Nuts and Seeds

Nuts and seeds have good fats and good, complex carbohydrates, and they even have pretty good proteins, which makes them an ideal food—if you don't have allergies. So if you're allergy free and you crave nuts, eat as many raw nuts and seeds as you want. Eventually, when you have taken in all the minerals, vitamins, and phytonutrients you need, you will start craving other foods, like fresh fruits and vegetables. You won't gain weight. In fact, in the long run, you will lose weight. Nuts can help reverse your diabetes—provided they're not covered in milk chocolate.

Nuts have several problems, the biggest being that they cause allergies and lectin intolerances. Intolerance means the nuts give you trouble, but don't kill you, whereas a really bad allergy and anaphylactic shock could kill you—with the tiniest amount of peanuts, for instance. Cashews especially are one of the causes of arthritis and back pain, so they should be eaten in small amounts only (two or three nuts), or not at all. (Did you know that they are in the same plant family as poison ivy?) And if you have rheumatoid arthritis, it is best to avoid cashews altogether.

To prevent most of the lesser "allergic" symptoms—bloating, joint swelling, back pain, itchy eyes, upset stomach, phlebitis—rotate nuts according to this plan.

MONDAY	Pecans, walnuts, hickories, butternuts
TUESDAY	Almonds, coconut, evening primrose seeds
WEDNESDAY	Flaxseeds, poppies, pumpkin seeds
THURSDAY	Brazil nuts, paradise nuts, cashews, pistachios, hemp seeds
FRIDAY	Hazelnuts, filberts, sunflower seeds
SATURDAY	Pine nuts, peanuts, chia seeds
SUNDAY	Sesame seeds, macadamia nuts, chestnuts, beech nuts, acorns

The idea is to have nuts and seeds from the same plant family just one day each week so you get a true rest on the other days of the week. If your allergy or intolerance symptoms increase while you are on the rotational diet, discontinue eating nuts.

- **Farm-raised and freshwater fish.** These are often more polluted and/or less nutritious than fish from the ocean.
- **Sodas and juices.** All regular versions of these are full of sugar, specifically fructose, which only raises your blood sugar. The diet varieties may sound healthier, but they aren't: They make your brain crave more unhealthy food and are clearly linked to our current wave of obesity.[27]
- **Salt.** Eating too much salt is unhealthy. The problem, however, is not so much sodium chloride itself, but rather the relative amount of salt compared with potassium, which is abundant in fruits and vegetables. If you salt your food, try to use an unadulterated sea salt or an herbed sea salt, and always drink enough fluids.
- **Alcohol.** All types of alcohol, but especially liquor and beer, are highly inflammatory and contain empty calories. Red wine contains the longevity molecule resveratrol; drink it moderately.

Green Is Life-Giving

On this Earth, plants came before people. With the "invention" of chlorophyll, life on Earth began to explode. Chlorophyll made it possible to harvest sunlight and turn it into sugars—fuel for animals and humans. It was the green revolution on Earth that brought us from a few bacteria and lichens to forests and prairies, and finally all insect and mammalian life. Where we see a green landscape, we feel relaxed, at home, and safe because humans cannot survive in places with eternal ice or bone-dry deserts. A green environment connotes water, a tolerable climate, and plants and animals that may nourish us.

The Goodness of Greens and Grasses

Besides chlorophyll, each plant also contains tens of thousands of chemical compounds, also called *phytochemicals*. These compounds are miniscule in weight compared to proteins, carbs, and fats and, therefore, were long overlooked by science. But each compound helps to repair, replace, and replenish

Nancy's Story

"I was diagnosed as a diabetic 2 years ago," says Nancy, who had been trying to control her blood sugar with her diet, since diabetes ran in her family. "I had felt that I was doomed, since my father, my father's mother, and also my mother's father all had diabetes."

After the diagnosis, Nancy says she struggled to keep her blood sugar stable. "I was able to keep my blood sugar low enough to stay off medication, but I wasn't on the right diet to keep it from going up and down."

Realizing that she had to change her diet in order to control her condition, Nancy decided to seek the advice of a Natural Medicine physician, who recommended that she follow an anti-inflammatory diet. Soon after, she noticed a change in her health.

"When I went to a Natural Medicine doctor and they told me that I needed to stop eating all sugar, wheat, oats, corn, dairy, and processed foods, things started improving drastically," she says. "I felt so much better! I wasn't getting the sugar 'highs and lows' anymore, and I wasn't getting shaky and anxious like I did before. I was even sleeping better at night, which helped me to have more energy and feel more in control of my body." But Nancy wasn't the only person who noticed a change in her body.

Six weeks after she began eating only anti-inflammatory foods, she was due for her 6-month blood sugar test. The results were astonishing: Nancy's A1c had dropped from 6.7 to 4.5! "My doctor asked me what I had done since I had been there 6 months earlier, because I had lost some weight and my reading was so much lower. The results were so amazing that they noted in my chart that I was no longer diagnosed as a diabetic!"

Based on her success, Nancy decided to make her new diet a new way of life—and she hasn't looked back. "I have been on this anti-inflammatory diet for almost 3 months now and have lost 15 pounds," she says, adding that she feels better than ever. "I finally have it mastered because I know what foods make my [blood] sugar go high. I know I can maintain this way of life for the rest of my life—so I can live forever!"

molecules your body has used; I call this the *goodness of greens and grasses*. Since the dawn of time, mankind has been living with plants and animals in close proximity—so close, in fact, that we have been eating them and sharing their molecules. Their molecules fit into your biochemistry and physiology like keys: They unlock your health because as plants and animals evolved, so did our bodies. Our cells need their cells' compounds in order to function well.

Since there are so many of these chemicals, not even the smartest doctor can figure them all out and hand them to you in pill form. Recent research has shown that phytochemicals may have anti-obesity properties, in addition to their anti-inflammatory nutrients.[28] So if you eat your vegetables, your body has the wisdom to determine what it needs and what it doesn't. It uses some molecules and discards others—and you don't even have to think about it. However, if you don't eat your vegetables, your body has no way to rebuild and repair its own cells. Ultimately, you'll experience nutritional deficiencies. These may be subtle at first, but after a while, they may develop into real disease.

Phytochemicals refer to the many compounds in a plant, while *phytonutrients* refer to those chemicals that we know will nourish our cells. Of course, there is no real difference between the two—in one case we know they are beneficial and in the other we haven't yet figured out all of their health benefits.

These small beneficial molecules help your cells function, much like vitamins do. But vitamins are only the tip of the iceberg; there are many phytonutrients in each plant. Their original purpose was to protect the cells from predators: Plants, storing tasty sugars and starches for the next season, are always in danger of being eaten—not only by humans, but also by animals and germs. So these clever plants protect themselves by producing phytochemicals that are poisonous to animals and germs. But if they're poisonous to animals, how are they safe—and even nutritious—for humans to eat? For millions of years, plants have produced those pesty little molecules to avoid being eaten. But humans ate some of the plants and their poisons anyway and learned to deal with—and even thrive on—them! Now phytonutrients, in one sense, are still poisons. But they have become necessary for our health. So phytonutrients are plant poisons originally manufactured for defense, but then adapted by our bodies for healthy function.

Of all the phytonutrients, the ones in the *polyphenol* group have garnered special attention because flavonoids belong in this group. Flavonoids are antioxidants that give color to your foods. *Oxidants* are free radicals roaming and creating inflammation and mischief in your body. *Antioxidants* bind oxidants with them, rendering them harmless and preventing diseases and premature aging. The truth is, vitamins alone are just not enough: One study found that only 0.4 percent of the antioxidant activity of an apple came from its vitamin C content—the rest came from polyphenols and flavonoids![29] And research has shown that including antioxidant phytonutrients in your diet can reduce your risk of developing type 2 diabetes.[30] It is not that vitamins are overrated, it's that phytonutrients are underrated.

Healing Greens

When shopping in your local supermarket for bitter, dark green vegetables, stock up on these diabetes-fighting foods.

- Amaranth
- Arugula
- Beet greens
- Bok choy
- Cabbages (all of them!)
- Chard
- Collard greens
- Dandelion
- Dinosaur kale (also called lacinato kale)
- Endive
- Escarole
- Kale
- Kohlrabi greens
- Lettuce
- Mâche (also called rapunzel, or corn salad)
- Mizuna
- Mustard greens
- Radicchio (this is the *red* green!)
- Spinach
- Watercress

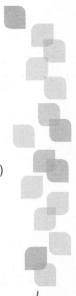

New greens are showing up all the time at farmers' markets and health food stores. Look around and try different greens for more adventurous eating!

There are other important groups of phytonutrients as well, including *terpenes, betalains, organosulfides,* and *indoles.* Terpenes, like the beta-carotene in carrots and lycopene in tomatoes, give yellow and orange color to your food. Betalains are responsible for the red color in beets and chard. Organosulfides are the colorless compounds that make all cabbages such great cancer fighters. Indoles help garlic fight bacteria and fungi, and even heart disease—similar to the actions of related compounds in cabbages. Scientists are finding new beneficial compounds all the time. But the good news is that you don't have to know their chemical structures or biochemical functions: If you simply eat your veggies, you'll reap their benefits.

Research has shown that incorporating phytonutrients into your diet is essential to losing weight and reversing the chronic inflammation that causes and maintains your diabetes.[31] While some phytonutrients may come from animals that eat plants, most come directly from the plants themselves. Vegetables have the highest density of phytonutrients, and a good sign of healthy nutrients is a slightly bitter taste. Yes, bitter vegetables are good for you!

Bitter Is Better

Because they contain healthy phytonutrients that work against inflammation in your body, you should eat a variety of vegetables every single day. But certain vegetables provide more anti-inflammatory punch than others: the bitter ones. When selecting your food, focus on choosing fresh, bitter, dark green vegetables, which contain more phytonutrients than any other plants.

You may not like the taste of bitter vegetables, but here's a surprise for you: Life was never supposed to be sweet. Our ancestors ate bitter vegetables all the time, until only a few generations ago. That's when homemade herbal bitters (alcoholic extractions of bitter herbs) were served before a meal, or brought out after a rich meal—the most famous being Swedish Bitters and angostura, which was commonly used in cocktails. But in these modern times, we favor sweets above all other tastes, and consequently, digestive problems are increasing.

The Bitter Principle

Bitter vegetables increase digestive juices, which helps you digest heavy meals.[32] Researchers have found taste receptors for bitter flavors not only on human tongues, but also in human guts. When stimulated, those receptors propel digestive matter forward. By digesting food quickly, our overstuffed stomachs feel relief faster. Bitter vegetables also shorten bowel transit time and prevent constipation. And according to a 2011 study, bitter receptors have recently even been found in lung tissue: They open up airways and might someday be used against asthma.[33] It seems that bitter medicines were always used against infections: Quinine against malaria, aloe against infected wounds, berberine (from goldenthread) against intestinal infections, and the "King of Bitter"—*Andrographis paniculata*—against colds. In addition to targeting inflammation, these greens prevent cancer and promote heart health, better vision,[34-36] and overall health in your immune system.

Bitter vegetables can heal your body. So we have to rediscover the bitter principle and use it when preparing our meals. Our lives have become too sweet, too cloying, too weak—and ultimately we've become too obese and too diabetic. And did I mention that bitter foods can be delicious? Bitter, leafy greens taste great when simmered in a little water with olive oil, garlic (fresh or dried), salt, and pepper!

The Superfoods Myth . . . Debunked!

You have read and heard it so often: "The 10 Best Foods" or "The 5 Best Fruits." Some of the lists contain meritable foods, often chosen based on their antioxidant contents. The usual suspects are almonds, avocados, beans, blueberries (all berries, really), broccoli, cinnamon, spinach, and walnuts. And there is nothing wrong with these foods. But the concept of "superfoods" is all wrong.

If you eat the same "superfood" again and again, you have a higher chance of developing an allergy to it or ingesting the same pollutants again and again. And you could even overdo it on some phytonutrients and become deficient in others. The goal is to eat a wide variety of meats, fish, and vegetables, preferably local and in season. So instead of focusing on specific "superfoods," focus on incorporating many different foods—especially vegetables—into your diet. Rotate what you eat, and savor eating foods that are in season.

Beyond Vegetables

My mantra is "Vegetables, vegetables, vegetables"; without inflammation-fighting vegetables, there is no health. If you picture your plate as three-quarters full with vegetables, you have another quarter to fill, which should be divided equally into protein and complex carbohydrates like whole grains and legumes. But what about *fat*? Most of your daily fat ration goes into the cooking of vegetables in olive oil; some fats also come with meats, fish, and eggs, and their preparation.

Eating Macronutrients

The discussion of *micronutrients* made it clear why vegetables should be your number one choice for healthy eating: They provide the "goodness of greens and grasses." But we should not overlook *macronutrients*: carbohydrates, proteins, and fats. They, of course, make up the bulk of your calories—and the bulk of your belly, if you are not careful. Macronutrients are inexpensive fillers, in the first place, and—if you let food manufacturers manipulate your taste buds—they can be coffin fillers, too. Therefore, we need to know more about macronutrients and which choices are best to aid in your fight against diabetes.

Proteins

You need proteins in your diet so that your body does not start to digest its own muscles. When most of us think of protein, we automatically think of *meat*. Or *fish*. Or *eggs*. But these are not the only sources of protein: Nuts, grains, legumes, mushrooms, and pseudograins like quinoa and amaranth are also good sources. However, meat, fish, and eggs contain a full set of amino acids (the building molecules of proteins) and valuable vitamin B_{12} that isn't typically found in plants, unless they are fermented. And since the human body has lost the ability to manufacture vitamin B_{12}, we have to get it from our food, which means you need to keep modest amounts of meat, fish, and eggs in your diet.

While some plants contain iron (essential for building blood), they provide much less than red meats readily offer. For all of these reasons, being a raw foodie, fruitarian, vegetarian, or vegan is no long-term nutritional solution.

All, however, are excellent cleansing diets for a month or two, when you come off the SAD. Just be careful to avoid a common pitfall of adapting a vegetarian diet for good: While pizza, doughnuts, muffins, and ice cream are definitely vegetarian foods, they don't contain any healthy cells or phytonutrients. A truly balanced meal has vegetables, fruit, healthy starches, good fats, and proteins.

Eating in Season

See the list below to determine which fruits and vegetables you might find in your produce aisle or garden each season to get the most benefits from fresh foods. The list is not exhaustive, so be sure to look around!

- **Winter:** From storage: broccoli, Brussels sprouts, cabbages, cauliflower, celeriac, celery, cranberries, kale, leeks, mâche (rapunzel), parsnips, potatoes, red beets, rutabaga, winter squash, turnips.

- **Spring:** apples, artichoke, arugula, asparagus, chard, fava beans, fiddleheads, kitchen herbs, lettuce, mâche (rapunzel), parsnips, peas, radish, rhubarb, scallions, spinach, spring garlic, spring onions, stinging nettle.

- **Summer:** arugula, asparagus, blackberries, black currants, blueberries, broccoli, cantaloupes, carrots, celery, chard, cherries, corn, cucumber, eggplant, garlic, spring garlic, gooseberries, green beans, kale, kitchen herbs, kohlrabi, leeks, melons, spring onions, peaches, pears, peas, plums, potatoes, radishes, raspberries, red beets, rhubarb, stinging nettles, strawberries, summer squash, winter squash, tomatoes, turnips.

- **Fall:** arugula, broccoli, Brussels sprouts, cantaloupes, carrots, cauliflower, celeriac, celery, chard, chicories, cranberries, cucumber, eggplant, escarole, garlic, grapes, green beans, kale, kitchen herbs, kohlrabi, leeks, melons, onions, parsnips, peas, peaches, pears, plums, potatoes, pumpkin, radishes, red beets, rutabaga, spring onions, stinging nettles, summer squash, winter squash, tomatoes, turnips.

How Much Protein?

Presently, there is a heated debate between vegetarians and vegans on one side and omnivores and meat eaters on the other side: Do we need meat in our diets? Because we need to repair our muscles, I come down on the omnivore side: We do need meat, the most complete source of amino acids. But we do not need huge amounts. How much is enough? Luckily, you are carrying around the perfect measuring tool wherever you go: The palm of your hand (width, breadth, and thickness) is a perfect measure of your daily meat allowance (fish and eggs included). If you are a bulky construction worker, your hand might be large. If you are a tiny writer, you obviously need less, as your hand is smaller. Now, this palm-size piece of protein is enough for the whole day—it is the combined size of all the meat, fish, and eggs you should eat that day. So if you down half a dozen eggs for breakfast, that's it—you've certainly had your share for the day, and probably more. Try to avoid eating too much protein because it can cause constipation, gallbladder inflammation (cholecystitis), loss of bone mass (osteoporosis/osteopenia), kidney stones, premature aging, and high blood pressure (hypertension).

Choosing Your Proteins

So which source of protein is best? For the longest time, I favored fish over meat because many studies told us that heart disease was related to red meats and animal fats and other studies touted the benefits of fish oil–rich ocean fish. But recently, fish seems more and more polluted and grass-fed organic meats are more readily available, appearing in the butcher aisles. In the end, your health depends upon the health of the animal you eat—and what that fish or animal ate, and how polluted and unnatural its environment was during its lifetime. Again, we are returning to the goodness of greens and grasses—now viewed from the animals' side. The closer the animal lived to an ideal lifestyle, the healthier its flesh will be. The best meats to eat for protein are animals that were grass fed because they became healthy by eating the same phytonutrients your cells need in order to function. For example, did you know that the meat that comes from outdoor-ranging animals has much higher levels of vitamin A than meat from indoor-kept livestock?[37] If you give it some thought, it makes sense: They graze under the sun all day and it shows up in their flesh, just as good food and daily walks will show up in your flesh, skin, hair, brain, and so on. But as you know, there are more sources of protein than just meat and fish. So take a look at the comprehensive list of protein sources available to you.

- Fish should not be farm-raised. Ocean fish are better for you than freshwater fish because of their higher omega-3 contents. And small fish are better to eat than big fish because small fish eat chlorophyll-rich plankton, whereas larger fish eat smaller fish, thus removing themselves even further from the goodness of greens, while also accumulating environmental poisons like mercury and pesticides.

- Lobsters, shrimp, prawns, and crabs are usually scavengers, also called detritivores or bottom feeders, which tells you that they are foraging on dead matter—nothing green. This is why their fats are not as healthy as fish oil and why you should eat them only occasionally.

- Mussels are mollusks and filter eaters—they filter plankton and phytoplankton from the water, which places them in the "goodness of greens and grasses" category. But mussels can be contaminated by human waste, pollutants, and algae, so get them from a reliable source.

- Squid (calamari) eat everything, it seems, so we should classify them as omnivores and eat them only occasionally.

- Abalone and sea urchins (uni) eat kelp, a type of seaweed, so they're healthy additions to your diet. But severe restrictions apply for harvesting this endangered abalone, so you may find that it's not always available.

- Snails are herbivores and have been a source of good proteins in times of famine. The French eat them in garlic butter as a delicacy called *escargots*.

- Red meats should come from animals that have eaten grass, have spent their lives in a pasture, and have not been treated with hormones, antibiotics, or other drugs. In a pinch, lamb is usually the least adulterated meat, even in a normal supermarket, because lambs stay out in the pasture their whole lives, without extra feed, hormones, and antibiotics.

- Game is the perfect meat. For reasons that elude me, it is forbidden to sell or buy game meat that is caught in the wild. Historically, fear of diseases acquired from wild meats was the reason. At a time when our commercial meat is laced with *E. coli* and other germs, that seems an out-of-touch decision. One can buy farm-raised game, which is inspected and certified. But anything that has been fed on a farm is not in its primal state anymore.

- Pork is "the other white meat," according to a popular advertisement. A pig is an omnivore, eating just about everything you put in front of it. So it is removed from the goodness of greens and grasses and should not be eaten on a regular basis. That said, if you're traveling and your choices are limited, go ahead and allow yourself to have some bacon. It isn't very processed and is definitely a better option than sugary cereal or pancakes with syrup.

- Poultry should be raised outside and should eat grass, weeds, and grubs, with little extra feed. We tend to think that the white meats of chicken and turkey are superior, but they are not. Darker meat contains more fat (and, therefore, is more satisfying) and more iron, which the human body needs. (Some iron can be assimilated from vegetables, but in smaller quantities.)

- Eggs should come from free-ranging hens who forage on grasses and grubs, with little extra feed. These eggs have more omega-3s in the yolks than commercial eggs do. The white of an egg is all protein. Make sure you stick to eating real eggs—not artificial egg substitutes.

- Deli meats, cured meats, canned "construction" meats (like Spam and corned beef), and sausages should not be part of your daily fare because they actually contain few real chunks of flesh, which isn't healthy for you. Avoid these meats unless you know a farmer who makes his own sausage.

- Tofu is the curd of soybeans. The protein-rich pulp is curdled and then formed into a firm block. From a health standpoint, tofu is not living up to its reputation. It is an industrial product—anything that comes in a perfect square can't be natural. (American cheese should have taught us that.) In the kitchen, tofu is versatile and cheap, but that's about it. Soy is touted as a phytoestrogen, but many other legumes are, as well. Rotating your beans and lentils would be far healthier for you (and the planet) than eating processed soy. Unprocessed soy, however, is rather unpalatable. And soy allergies are common, causing skin problems, arthritis, and indigestion.

- Tempeh, originally from Indonesia, is a better soy product—but stick with the organic kind. Fermentation makes tempeh more easily digestible and healthier than tofu, and its tightly packed cakes of whole soybeans promote bowel health and provide vitamins. Tempeh is an excellent source of protein, as it contains the complete amino acids essential for humans.

- **Tofu burgers and veggie burgers** are inherently processed, inferior foods, even if they claim they are vegetarian or vegan. Opt instead for small hamburgers made at home from grass-fed organic meat.

A rule of thumb: Most people eat too much protein, having it with nearly every meal. To reduce this, try to have a vegetarian dinner without meat, poultry, or fish three times a week. Mushrooms and eggs are good substitutes when you're going meatless.

The Proteins in Dairy: Helpful or Harmful?

Studies have shown that milk and dairy products give us proteins, but these proteins are both inflammatory and allergenic.[38] Dairy products also provide fats (which are rich in calories) and milk sugar (lactose), to which many people are intolerant. The milk industry has drilled it into us that dairy is health food, but what should we believe? Milk is a calorie-rich food designed by Nature for calves. Apart from the inflammatory proteins, milk from the typical dairy cow is loaded with pus—an article too unappetizing to drink or give to your children. Cheese—real cheese, like a French Brie or a Dutch Gouda or a Swiss cheese with holes—contains healthy bacteria, that's true. But American "cheese" cannot even claim the health benefits of bacteria because it is just a chemical concoction of milk solids, fats, artificial colors, and flavorings—plus large amounts of salt. So my best advice on dairy is: Stay away from this addictive substance!

Fats

You can keep your body supplied with short-term fuel (glucose) all the time. But if you do this, by around age 40 you will have exhausted your pancreas's ability to supply your body with insulin, which means you will eventually develop type 2 diabetes. So it's better to stock up on some long-term fuel, namely fat. Fat has such a bad reputation that you don't even want to think *fat* and *my body* at the same time. But the truth is we are carrying a lot of fat around: Roughly 20 percent of a man's body mass is fat, and about 25 percent of a woman's.

Fats are important fuel for your body, and they come in all forms. The scientific name of fats is lipids—oils are liquid lipids, fats are solid lipids. You may not be aware that fats are one of the storage forms of sugars and that they will be reverted to sugar when your body needs the fuel. Nobody wants to be fat, but you need to eat fats for future energy and to perform several important tasks in your body. Fat is not the villain it is made out to be, but you have to learn which fats are good for you and which are not.

It turns out that saturated fats aren't all as unhealthy as you have been told. There are good and bad saturated fats. For that reason, in my kitchen I use coconut oil, olive oil, and ghee (clarified butter)—and, when I can get my hands on it, duck fat. Long ago, I found out that *my* body and brain need lots of fats to function; you might need less. Find out what *you* need. Are you always hungry and irritable? Or are you constantly cold when other people find the environment toasty? If so, you may need more fat in your diet. Bear in mind that about one-quarter of your weight is made up of fats,[39] so your body needs them. Every cell in your body is surrounded by a fatty cell wall. And if you don't replace the old walls with good new ones, your cell walls become leaky, or rigid, or both, making you sick and/or old. Fats are also an important part of messenger molecules (hormones), carrying information throughout your body. Without fat, those molecules are silenced. And if you scrimp on good fats, you hurt your fattiest organ—your brain—most of all.[40]

Most fats from plants are healthy when they are freshly pressed. But they bind to oxygen in the air rather quickly and become rancid. Rancidity not only renders good oils useless, it also turns the oils into inflammatory poison: They have become oxidants, instead of antioxidants. Because fresh oils turn rancid so easily, food manufacturers have discovered *partial hydrogenation*: the process of taking perishable oils and "hydrogenating" them, giving them a long shelf life. Unfortunately, they also took all the goodness out of the oils in the process, turning them harmful—and, in essence, giving Americans the epidemic of heart disease. Heart disease and hardening of the arteries did not come from saturated fats, but from hydrogenated fats, which are also called trans fats.

Trans fats are also built up as soon as you overheat fats in the process of frying or, worse, deep-frying. That's why coconut oil (virgin and, if possible, organic) is the preferred fat for pan-frying: It has the highest heating point before it denaturizes. And as we discussed, high heat—from baking, broiling, frying, roasting, and so on—creates dangerous advanced glycation end products (AGEs), which promote aging, cancer, and diabetes.[41] So these cooking methods shouldn't be used often.

Every plant food (vegetable, fruit, herb, legume, or grain) should be served with a little fat so that you can absorb the fat-soluble compounds like vitamins A, D, E, and K. If you eat your salad without fat, your body cannot absorb the salad's wonderful vitamins. We typically eat salads correctly (topped with some type of oil), but nobody eats an apple with some fat. An apple and an egg—that would be more like it!

Carbohydrates

Carbohydrates fall into two groups: simple and complex. Simple carbohydrates are milled and refined, and those we call sugars and starches don't contain any cells at all. Starches are the storage form of sugars, all linked in long chains. But they're digested in the blink of an eye, and then they become sugars again, flooding your system and creating havoc and diabetes.

Complex carbohydrates still contain the original plant cells and, therefore, nourish your body: Beans and lentils are examples, as are sweet potatoes and red beets. Before you can digest the starches in a sweet potato or red beet, your digestive juices have to crack open every single cell wall in your food. And this is the natural process of slow digestion for which our bodies are designed. Modern food manufacturing, however, put sugar on the tips of our tongues, and now we don't want to be bothered with the cooking, chewing, and digesting anymore. But to restore your health and reverse the inflammation in your body, you have to return to eating the complex carbohydrates that are in every plant food, including fruit, vegetables, legumes, whole grains, nuts, herbs, and seaweeds.

The more sugars and starches a plant has, the more dangerous that plant is for diabetics. This is why I emphasize vegetables over fruit, temperate fruit over tropical fruit, and aboveground vegetables over root vegetables. But all of those sweet and starchy plants still contain whole cells and abundant good phytonutrients, so eat them—but in moderation!

How to Read Labels

Food manufacturers are not concerned about your health. Regardless of what they advertise, don't be fooled by claims that you will lose weight, look beautiful forever, or miraculously feel better by eating a specific product. Here are some commonly used terms often associated with "healthy" food.

- **Low-fat or partially hydrogenated.** If a food item is intended to be stored in a warehouse or supermarket, the fats in it have to be partially hydrogenated to give the product a long shelf life. Hydrogenating makes an unhealthy fat out of a healthy fat—like sunflower oil in "healthy" margarines. Your body needs fats to function properly, but *good* fats!

- **No fat.** When you see this label on a product that contains grains like wheat or corn, it means that this product is made from starches that contain absolutely no healthy parts of the original grains. Every single kernel that was ever grown contains fat to nourish the plant that is supposed to grow from this little kernel. If milling removes the outer hulls and only leaves the inner starch, you get "fat free"—but you also get no fiber, no vitamins, no healthy fats and oils, and absolutely no phytonutrients.

- **Natural.** This label means that the original ingredients have, at some point, been grown—regardless of how many "refining" processing steps have adulterated the product since then. According to this definition, sugar qualifies as "natural" even if it has none of the vitamins, minerals, and phytonutrients contained in the original sugarcane. "Natural" is misleading to consumers, and it definitely does not mean that the plant was grown under organic conditions.

Sugars

After dairy, sugars are the most damaging food ingredients for diabetics. Sugar has calories but no nutritional value: It doesn't provide any healthy chemicals that build or repair your cells. Plus, sugar robs you of essential B vitamins. Sugar is addictive for many people, so avoid it whenever possible.

A short study of a small sample of people showed that honey compares well on all sugar and inflammation-measuring parameters, including blood sugar, blood lipids, C-reactive protein, and homocysteine.[42] And ghrelin

- **Gluten-free.** While this label tells you that the product does not contain wheat, rye, or barley, it does not mean that this product is necessarily healthy. Most gluten-free store-bought baked goods contain too much sugar, and they contain mostly empty starches and calories. Gluten-free can, therefore, be a trap for diabetics. Also, since most gluten-free products were processed in factories, they can be slightly contaminated with gluten-containing grains. For most gluten-intolerant people, that does not pose a problem. But for those who have a gluten allergy in the narrow medical sense of "allergy," the tiniest amounts of gluten could trigger a reaction or even anaphylactic shock.

- **Roasted.** When this appears on a package containing nuts, it likely means that the nuts were old (as roasting hides rancidity) and that they have lost most of their healthy omega-3 fats through heating. Be aware that by law, all Californian almonds have to be irradiated—and it isn't required to be mentioned on the package.

- **Evaporated cane juice.** This is a fancy word for "refined sugar."

- **No label.** If a product doesn't have a label but has a barcode, take note of the five-number code the cashier types into the register. It gives you two important pieces of information: If the first digit is a 9, the product is organic. If the first digit is an 8, the product is genetically modified (contains genetically modified organisms, or GMOs) and is certainly not organic.

levels respond better to honey than to dextrose or sucrose. But for a diabetic, the health benefits of honey might be too small to measure against the risk that she will never lose her sweet tooth. Therefore, I don't recommend that diabetics use honey as a sweetener—however, if you do want to sin, it is the right sugar to sin with!

I should note that the American Diabetes Association (ADA) thinks

The Glycemic Index versus Phytonutrients

You may be wondering how the glycemic index (GI) factors into following an anti-inflammatory, phytonutrient-rich diet. Carbohydrates spike your blood sugar, and the glycemic index ranks food items by assessing two aspects of carbohydrates:

1. The amount of carbohydrates in a certain food

2. How fast those carbohydrates turn up in your blood to elevate your blood sugar

The second aspect depends on several factors, namely the presence of fiber, which binds sugars so that they are slowly released into your bloodstream, and cell walls, which need to be digested before the sugars can be released. Additional factors, like how much fat or vinegar is in the food (both of these also slow the release of sugars), should also be considered.

The glycemic index gives you a quick overview of how "sugary" foods are and tells you to avoid the ones that rank high. This ranking was determined by feeding healthy volunteers a specific food and watching how much their blood glucose spiked afterward. But one problem with the GI is that foods might look healthier on paper than they are in reality. For starters, the GI is a list of "foods" put together by nutritionists who are thinking in terms of modern branded food items you can buy in a supermarket or convenience store. You and I already know that a convenience store barely offers anything nutritious. And to add insult to injury, they calibrated the whole glycemic index to white bread, which means that every food item is compared to an artificial "food" that gives you absolutely no people should be able to indulge in a bit of sugar, but this thinking doesn't take sugar addiction into account. And they slyly add that, of course, sugar consumption has to be combined with more exercise. The ADA also thinks that "starchy foods are part of a healthy meal plan."[43] Starch is cheap, that much can be said for it, but this advice could be deadly for diabetics, especially with white starches.

nourishment—only calories. (By the way, this cardboard "food" is still served to patients in hospitals, regardless of whether or not they have diabetes.)

Physicians issue warnings about, for instance, red beets and cherries, claiming that they are too sweet and, therefore, dangerous and should not be eaten. However, the doctors usually don't warn patients about the dangers of consuming white bread, which has a higher GI and none of the good chemical compounds found in cherries and red beets.[44] White bread has no nutritional value, whereas every single plant is already fortified with all of the phytonutrients that have been nourishing our bodies throughout history—at least until factory food was invented in the 19th century.

While the glycemic index provides some useful information, its usefulness is limited. If you look through the hundreds of glycemic index lists that are readily available these days, they typically compare a slew of bad foods—as if it matters that a Chocolate Raspberry Zing Bar, at 47, fares better than a Milky Way Lite Bar, at 62! Instinctively you know that both are bad for you, whatever the numbers say.

If you find that a plant has a high GI rating—and it is a whole plant food—it simply means you need to practice portion control. For example, have your 10 cherries—just don't eat the whole bag. This way, you won't miss out on all the good anti-diabetic compounds and antioxidants the cherries contain.

Following the glycemic index is not the answer when you are choosing a food. Freshness is what counts! Put meals together that are *nourishing,* because it's only when you focus on a diet rich in anti-inflammatory foods that you can begin to cure your diabetes.

Cooking Your Anti-Inflammatory Food

Cooking is essential because while it can destroy some valuable nutrients in food, it also makes others more available. For this reason, I am not a proponent of the raw food movement—although a nice salad, green smoothie, and piece of fresh fruit here and there are a good idea. And naturally, we tend to eat more raw food in summer and cook more in winter. Again, there's not one rule for every time and every person, but here are some guidelines for choosing your cooking methods.

Microwaves. When you microwave a food, you lose about two-thirds of the polyphenols[45]—the wonderful plant compounds that make your vegetables so nourishing. Other methods of cooking destroy some polyphenols, too, but not as many—usually between 30 and 50 percent total. So when you're cooking vegetables, try to use your stovetop or oven so that you're getting as many health benefits from your food as possible.

Indoor grills. I would not recommend using indoor electric grills because the nonstick Teflon griddles create toxic fluorocarbon gases when heated. There are versions without Teflon, but they're more expensive. Another reason I don't recommend this kind of kitchen appliance: In most cases it takes less time to grill a piece of meat than it does to clean and cook vegetables, so you end up eating meat too often—and grilled meat is high in AGEs.

Outdoor grills. Like all high-heat cooking methods, grilling creates trans fats and AGEs. Use the grill only very occasionally—like on the Fourth of July!

Slow cookers. These generally make wonderful one-pot dinners. You can set them on low in the morning (make sure they are attached to a circuit breaker!) and find your dinner ready when you come home—perfect for those who work all day.

Clay pots. These braise meat (through slow cooking) wonderfully—I own three different sizes and use them mostly for festive meats on special occasions. One advantage is that this cooking process is faster than on the stove. More importantly, you never have to baste the meat. It always comes out crisp and juicy. The clay pots are not cheap, but if you don't drop them and you remember to keep them out of the dishwasher, they'll last forever.

Return to the Family Meal

Once you understand that you cannot be healthy while living on ready-made foods, you will want to cook for yourself and your family. Contrary to popular belief, it does not take much time to cook. And by throwing out dinner as family time, people are abandoning one important family-building tool: To eat and laugh and talk about the day and the world every day at the dinner table shapes the character of your child like nothing else will. Return to the family dinner table (and to a family breakfast). What could be more important than the health of your family?

Rules for Eating

You now know which foods you should avoid eating, which foods you should eat to fight your inflammation, and how your meals should be prepared. But here are a few simple rules to help you stay on track and ultimately get the most out of each meal.

1. **Never go hungry!** It's important to make sure you're full and satisfied at the end of each meal. This will go a long way toward helping you to turn down any "fake" foods you may encounter throughout the day.

2. **Be fresh.** Everything you eat should have grown somewhere and should have cells. So whenever you get ready to eat, ask yourself whether your food is fresh or contains preservatives. If it's the latter, don't eat it.

3. **Watch your portions.** Your meal should fill your dinner plate. If you feel that this is too much for your size and energy expenditure, try using a smaller plate.

4. **Eliminate snacks.** There is no snacking after the first 4 weeks. After the first month, your body will no longer be in the cycle of high sugar spikes and hypoglycemic episodes. But during these first 4 weeks, choose from the healthy snack list on the next page.

5. **Take a break after dinner.** No eating between dinner and breakfast at all. Exception: If you are still taking insulin or diabetes medications,

other rules apply. But—even then—stay away from sweets, cheese, crackers, and again, choose from the healthy snack list below.

6. **Drink clean.** Avoid beverages that contain calories; instead, stick to water and herbal, green, or black tea.

Do You Need a Snack?

Snacking is a bad idea because few people fare well on the "eat-more-but-smaller meals" advice. Instead, they tend to eat more meals, but the sizes of the meals remain large. If you find that you absolutely need a snack, make sure that you're eating the right snacks at the right times. Sit down to eat, pay attention to your food, and do not eat on the go, because then the choices are often bad. And avoid eating at night, so that your body has a chance to heal and repair from the day before. Here are some options for healthy, filling snacks.

- **Avocado.** This is the perfect snack fruit, with protein, fat, and flavor! Eat it as is, or make guacamole with a small fresh onion, a tomato, a bit of olive oil, pepper, and salt.

- **Dark chocolate.** Snack on a small milk-free piece—preferably with no added sugar.

- **Dried fruit.** This is a great on-the-go snack. Eat a small handful of raisins, dried blueberries, dried raspberries (nothing with extra sugar!), or dried apple pieces. But go easy on dried fruit if your blood sugar is still high.

- **Egg salad.** Best if made with good mayonnaise, try it sprinkled with chives or other herbs from the garden or grocery store. A plain egg also makes a great snack.

- **Fresh, unroasted and untoasted nuts and seeds.** Options like hazelnuts, walnuts, pecans, Brazil nuts, almonds, sunflower seeds, and sesame seeds are filling snacks.

- **Fresh fruit.** You can take a piece of fruit like an apple or a pear every-where, since it does not need much planning and preparing. Combine a piece of fruit with nuts for some added healthy fat.

- **Hot chocolate.** Try a teaspoon of sugar-free cacao powder in a cup that's filled up two-thirds with hot water and one-third with

Cell-ebrate!

We have talked so much about healthy nutrition and how it can improve your diabetes. What we have not mentioned enough is how good you will feel if you pamper yourself with cells and freshness. You will wake up in the morning with energy and without the usual aches and pains. Even

non-GMO unsweetened soymilk (or use hot water only). You can include stevia, but try to cut back on the amount you use each time to help get rid of your sweet tooth. This drink is a mild pick-me-up in the afternoon.

- **Hummus.** While this can be a great snack, make sure it doesn't contain preservatives—just chickpeas, sesame seeds, garlic, and salt. Buy a small amount and eat it shortly after purchase.

- **Olives.** A few olives make a great snack to keep you satisfied throughout the afternoon and until dinnertime.

- **Popcorn.** A fun snack, popcorn is reasonably healthy and cheap, but pop it yourself from organic kernels with a splash of olive oil. If you have a popper, fine; otherwise use a pot with a sturdy lid over high heat. The popcorn is done as soon as the popping gets spaced out. After all the popping has stopped, let the lid stay on for at least another 5 minutes without having a peek! While popcorn is high in fiber, it's also high in white starch, so eat it sparingly. It's not a staple for every day—shoot for once or twice a month.

- **Sardines.** Whether from the can with a bit of pepper and salt or as a fish salad with a small amount of chopped onion, half an apple, and some dill, sardines can give you some protein at any time of day. Add a few nuts or seeds for texture.

- **Seaweed.** When toasted in sesame oil, seaweed can be very tasty. You can also munch on untoasted seaweed—it's a bit less tasty, but still healthful.

- **Trail mix.** Make sure to create your own trail mix to avoid the processed particles in prepackaged mixes. You'll be sure to get the health benefits of fresh nuts, as well.

more important (and surprising), you will start your day with new purpose and vitality. Where before you needed rest and downtime to recover—and more and more of it—now you will feel as if you want to tackle all kinds of endeavors and pursuits. This will be your new *you*, the one you were meant to be all along. Just think what the world would look like if we all always operated at our best, at full speed and with abundant strength and purpose to really pursue our happiness. It is what's

Tips for Affordable Food Shopping

Do you think a $1 burger or a bag of potato chips with a bottle of soda is a cheap meal? It's not cheap if you get depressed, achy, and listless from what you are eating! It's not cheap if you consider the health costs down the line from arthritis, diabetes, high blood pressure, cancer, and depression. It's not cheap if you consider the cost of constantly needing larger sizes of clothing—and the human misery that comes with that.

The government subsidizes corn, soy, wheat, and dairy, which is why manufacturers use those ingredients excessively and push them on customers. But they are not healthy. Be the change you want to see in the world, and buy healthy foods. Below are some tips to help you shop affordably.

- Most fresh items in season are reasonably priced. Good food *can* be inexpensive.
- Buy staples like lentils and chickpeas in ethnic stores. Also, these stores often sell dried herbs in bulk.
- If you can't afford to buy everything organic, it is more important to get organic meat, poultry, and eggs than to eat organic fruits and vegetables. Also, try to buy wild-caught fish.
- Never go shopping with a set recipe in your mind; buy what is fresh, on sale, and organic, and then go home to figure out what you can make with your purchases.

promised to all of us and is achieved by so few. Think of what you want to do with your life; now you can finally rid your body of diabetes and reach for your dreams!

- Never go shopping hungry; you'll end up buying either more than you need or more of the wrong foods.

- In your fridge, line the vegetable crisper with paper towels; they absorb moisture and keep your veggies from rotting quickly.

- Fresh food spoils easily, so don't let it sit in the fridge—do something with it. All wilting veggies are still perfect for stir-fry or medley soup, for instance.

- Use what you have in different ways: The leftover bones from a turkey make a good soup or stock; use the beet roots *and* the greens (if they still look good); use leftovers for stews, soups, filled pastries, one-pot dinners, and more.

- Plan ahead to have leftovers of whatever you cook and prepare: Those will be your lunches during the coming week. Not buying from the vendor across the street will improve your health and your finances.

- Don't try to save money by forgoing fruits and vegetables; save money by questioning every item with a brand name, long shelf life, really funny or appealing ad on TV, or that comes in beautiful packaging, has words on its label that you can't pronounce, or contains ingredients your great-grandmother wouldn't have known.

Herbs
and Spices

∙∙

Nature grows an herb against each and every ill.

SEBASTIAN KNEIPP (1821–1897)

Now that you've learned the first component of your new lifestyle—eating anti-inflammatory foods—you're ready to take the next step toward reclaiming your health and curing your diabetes. And here's a bonus: You can make your new meals even healthier (and tastier, too!) while strengthening your fight against the diabetes-inducing inflammation in your body. How? Once again, we will look to Nature and whole plant foods.

The Importance of the Color Green

Green is the color of life, and we associate it with vegetables and health. But vegetables are not the only green plants that contain those healthy phytonutrients. Research has proven that you'll get even higher doses from herbs and spices, because they often come from environments (like the tropics or subtropics) that are hard on any individual species.[1] As a result, the plants have to work even harder to fight off predators, which causes them to build up high doses of phytochemicals that are healthy for us. But think of them as your new icing on the cake: Nobody would eat a whole jar of cinnamon in one session. Instead, we sprinkle these intense spices over our foods to enhance their benefits.

Alternative Medicine

Have you ever hesitated to tell your doctor that you take an herb? Or that you are trying a massage to help with your aches? Have you ever had a physician yell at you because you dared to mention an alternative method at all? I have been looking for gentle healing methods for more than 25 years now, and I am astonished when I still hear about such fossil physicians and incidents.

Why are herbal remedies still called *alternative*? There is nothing alternative about using healing foods and herbs to help patients, as they have been used throughout our evolution. And a new study has shown that overweight, underexercised physicians are utilizing fewer food and physical modalities to help their patients.[2] In practical terms, this means that overweight, underexercised physicians prescribe more medications.

In Europe, many alternative modalities such as herbal therapy, Natural Medicine, massage, acupuncture, yoga, relaxation, hydrotherapy, traditional Chinese medicine (TCM), Ayurvedic medicine, chiropractic, and biophysical medicine are considered mainstream, meaning health insurance pays for these services. A physician can pass an examination in a subspecialty in front of a board of peers to show his or her knowledge of these areas. In fact, I have done it—I became a physician for Natural Medicine in 1998. In the United States, we are still waiting for alternative specialty boards to become legal.

Are there quacks in alternative medicine? Sure there are. But they also exist within conventional medicine. The lack of communication between these two essential sides of medicine only perpetuates the shortcomings on both sides of the aisle.

Herbs as Medicine

Herbs and spices are packed with antioxidants and vitamins. Research has shown that when eaten, they decrease inflammation and eliminate the free radicals that hurt your cells.[3] And because the same biochemistry that governs your body is also at work in plants, herbs are perfect for healing (and they add taste and zest to your meals as well). For millions of years, we have coevolved with plants. And without those plants, we get sick.

Within a century, we moved from living off the land and thriving to becoming sick, overweight, and so depressed and anxious that the use of antidepressants has gone up 400 percent in the last 20 years.[4] We are sick because we are denied vital nutrients from our foods. While we can see some effects of our dietary choices (such as obesity), there are others we can't see: the unhappiness and multitude of illnesses that result from cell malnutrition. Eating vegetables, spices, and kitchen herbs will be your ticket to profound well-being.

But herbs can be a bit trickier to eat. You can really eat any vegetable you want without having to worry about experiencing side effects, but consuming medicinal plants requires some additional knowledge because they are more potent. In the past, women handed down this knowledge in their own households. But this practice was abandoned, for the most part. Now our generation is reclaiming this old wisdom—this time through modern books instead of ancestral teachings.

Synergy in Herbs

Synergy is the innate beauty in plant medicines: The whole plant works better than the individual parts. But since no one can patent a whole plant, manufacturers are not allowed to reap the profits. As a result, pharmaceutical firms try to either take out one component of a plant (the one they deem the "effective" part) or change one component chemically, so they can patent this as a new drug. (This is actually how many good drugs have been developed.) But when we neglect to use the whole plant, we are losing vital nutrients and health agents.

Synergy is one of the main reasons why herbs are so profoundly effective. The other reason is that plants are the keys to our ancient physiology: Plants and people developed together. Plant molecules are not new alien molecules our bodies can't recognize; they are old molecules that our bodies are very familiar with, so they can be happily incorporated into our old-fashioned metabolisms.

If a plant is toxic to us, it is only because the plant developed for that purpose. Whole plants are often less toxic than would be expected, because they provide counteracting "smoothing" ingredients that help us digest them. But medicinal plants also pose difficulties: The medicinal properties of harvested herbs will be stronger or weaker depending on when, where, and how the plant was grown and cut. And this is an obstacle for modern medicine, which requires predictable and reproducible products. For that purpose, herbs are sometimes "standardized": Different strength extractions are combined with certain key compounds so that the results are uniform. For example, St. John's wort had long been standardized to one of its "main" ingredients—until it became clear that it was not the "effective" one. Sometimes, it is hard to determine which elements are most beneficial in a plant that could contain more than 10,000 different chemical compounds.

The same is true for single compounds. For instance, scientists are still discovering new effects of taking aspirin, which has been on the market since 1899! If one single ubiquitous chemical is so hard to understand, just imagine how hard it is to understand all of the effects of a whole plant. Herbs require more knowledge and more experience to use than the other Essentials of Health. So for more difficult problems, you may find that you need the help of an herbalist or a doctor trained in Natural Medicine.

How to Use Herbs

To get you started, here are three ways to use herbs and spices.

1. **To add flavor, color, and healing ingredients to your meals.** Regardless of your food choice, it can be spruced up with herbs and spices: Vegetables, meat, fish, eggs—even a simple dessert—can be transformed into a piece of culinary art with a sprig of mint.

2. **Against a disease.** There is an herbal remedy for almost everything: when you get a cold, cut yourself, have a urinary tract infection, can't sleep, or are bothered by menopausal symptoms.

3. **As an adaptogen.** You are probably familiar with the use of herbs and spices in food. And maybe you've even taken a few herbs to combat specific ailments (such as drinking unsweetened cranberry juice to fight simple urinary tract infections, eating garlic to lower cholesterol, or taking a black cohosh supplement to relieve the symptoms of menopause). But have you ever heard of an herbal tonic? Tonics do not target a specific organ, but instead strengthen your overall health—especially your immune system and your nerves—over time.

The word *tonic* was not always associated with *gin*. In times before modern medicine, a tonic was used as a health-strengthening drink. It was prescribed to a child after he recovered from a severe fever, to a mother to help her recover after childbirth, to an elderly gentleman to keep up his stamina, or to a soldier who struggled after he came home from war. A tonic is not a placebo. Instead tonics, or *adaptogens*, as modern physicians call them, harness the nutrients of green herbs, berries, roots, mushrooms, and barks to restore a depleted body or mind. They also increase resistance to all kinds of diseases.[5] Luckily, you're not expected to mix your own tonics these days, as they are now available as drops or capsules at your local health food stores.

HERBS FOR TONICS

Look through the list on the next page and choose something that fits your needs. Take it religiously for a month or two and make sure to follow the dosage

Signs You May Need an Herbal Tonic

So how do you know which tonic you—or your doctor—should choose? Basically, you should choose the one that addresses any symptoms you may exhibit.

- Anxiety
- Chronic fatigue
- Convalescence
- Cravings for sugars and/or alcohol
- Emotional sensitivity
- Frequent colds and infections
- Generally feeling stressed-out and run-down
- Impatience

- Inability to concentrate
- Insomnia
- Insulin resistance
- Irritability
- Liver disease
- Moodiness
- Muscle weakness
- Poor nutrition
- Procrastination
- Toxic exposure

directions on the bottle. But discuss this with your physician, as adaptogens are potent and you may require guidance. Because some culinary herbs and medicinal herbs use the same common name, I've included the botanical names to help you discern which species you need.

- **Ashwaganda** (*Withania somnifera*) is an Indian herb used for its calming effect. This would be a good tonic if you are high-strung, anxious, irritable, and tend to have road rage. But make sure it isn't your thyroid that is hyper and sends you into a rage. As a nice side effect, ashwagandha lowers blood sugar.[6]

- **Astragalus** (*Astragalus membranaceus*) is a Chinese plant in the pea family. Its root counteracts weakness, fatigue, and low blood pressure. This root strengthens the *chi*, or life force, when taken in small doses over a long period of time. But it is powerful and may raise your blood pressure too high, so monitor yourself for headaches and nervousness when on this remedy. Traditionally used for diabetes, astragalus lowers insulin resistance and seems to help with a fatty liver.

- **Eleutherococcus** (*Eleutherococcus senticosus*) was originally used to combat chronic fatigue and enhance athletic performance. Newer studies have not been able to corroborate its effect on muscles and endurance, but it does work against depression and toward bringing hormones in balance,[7-8] so it is an adaptogen that I would recommend to a tired, depressed patient. For people with diabetes, its anti-inflammatory and lipid-lowering properties are of interest.[9]

- **Ginseng** (*Panax ginseng*) is a famous (and expensive) Chinese strengthening, anti-aging medicine. It's reserved for older populations as it is thought to be wasted on those younger than 50. It helps you lose weight by speeding up your metabolism but should be taken with caution as it can raise blood pressure and push your heart into overdrive, causing palpitations. Ginseng is popular because it's rumored to improve the sex lives of both genders, but diabetics might like its anti-hyperglycemic action.[10-11] But if you take it in one of the sugary solutions we often see in the market, it won't help your diabetes, so make sure you're using a natural form.

- **Jiao gu lan** (*Gynostemma pentaphyllum*) is another Chinese heal-all tonic; it's reputed to lower cholesterol and blood pressure, thus improving heart health. It supports your immune system and is often used alongside cancer treatments. Its anti-aging and sex-enhancing properties make it a favorite in China, but I mostly recommend it for its anti-diabetic qualities because it improves glycemic control.[12]

- **Licorice** (*Glycyrrhiza glabra*) is often taken for stomach ailments, but it is also a strengthening tonic. This herb is ideal for women with low estrogen, who are run-down, and who have signs of inflammation like diabetes, fatty liver, and arthritis. It also works well in men with problems along the hypothalamic-pituitary-adrenal axis, otherwise known as hormonal imbalances. Use caution when taking licorice, as some people develop high blood pressure. For that reason it is better to take DGL (deglycyrrhizinated) licorice when you take it for stomach problems. Recently, anti-diabetic substances called *amorfrutins* have been found in licorice root.[13]

- **Maitake** (*Grifola frondosa*) is a frilly, very large mushroom. Like all medicinal mushrooms, it enhances immune action. This one is also used to fight cancer and diabetes.[14]

- **Reishi** (*Ganoderma* spp.) is a group of medicinal Japanese tonic mushrooms famous for lowering blood pressure and—more relevant to our purpose here—blood sugar.[15-16] They are sometimes sold fresh in health food stores, but not quite as often as shiitake mushrooms.

- **Rhodiola** (*Rhodiola rosea*) is a beautiful Arctic plant in the same family as hens-and-chickens. Its well-known hardiness has been thought to be transferable to humans as a medicine. It lightens up your mood (but in certain people it can lighten it too much, leading to anxiety and mania) and fights fatigue and exhaustion. Rhodiola gives you antioxidants and protects your heart and nerves[17]—all helpful in people with diabetes. A related plant, *Rhodiola sacra*, is used in Arabic and Tibetan medicine for similar ailments and supports your mood, heart, and nerves.[18]

- **Sarsaparilla** (*Aralia nudicaule*) should not be confused with other plants called sarsaparilla. Native Americans used the roots for food during their long treks to a new summer or winter location. And it's one of the roots that went into the original root beer. I make teas consisting of this root, wild goldenrod, and a local spirea. This form of sarsaparilla has no apparent side effects.

- **Schizandra** (*Schisandra chinensis*) is used as an aphrodisiac in TCM.[19]

But more to the point, it has antihyperglycemic properties, and it is an effective medicine against the fatty liver that accompanies type 2 diabetes.[20–21]

- **Shiitake mushroom** (*Lentinula edodes*) contains the polysaccharide *lentinan*, which positively modulates your immune system.[22] Lentinan, unfortunately, is also the same compound that can give you an allergy, though this is extremely rare. While shiitake can lower blood sugar, it is traditionally used for stomach ailments and cancers.

- **Stinging nettle** *(Urtica urens, U. dioica)* is considered the most important herb in Europe because its root transforms the immune system.[23] The German Commission E approved the herb as therapy against inflammation and the root as therapy for prostate enlargement.[24] The whole plant contains marvelous nutrients. Besides giving you what you need in times of dearth, it also takes what you don't need: waste products and toxins. Nettle is the perfect gentle diuretic and cleanses the blood. Traditionally, it has been used to fight the effects of diabetes, perhaps for its detoxifying and anti-inflammatory actions. In a 2011 study, 50 men and women with type 2 diabetes participated in an 8-week double-blind trial to determine the effects of stinging nettle on inflammation. The intervention group received 100 milligrams of stinging nettle three times a day while the control group received a placebo. At the end of the study, the intervention group experienced a significant decrease in inflammatory markers over the control group.[25] The cleansing action leaves you feeling renewed and protects you from diseases, including cancer.[26] I grow this "weed" in my garden and use it as a dark green leafy vegetable that we enjoy until a hard frost kills the last shoots.

- **Suma** (*Pfaffia paniculata*) is used as a heal-all and tonic. Also known as Brazilian ginseng, it is relatively unknown in the West but has good potential: A study showed it has cancer-fighting properties.[27]

ANTI-DIABETIC HERBS AND SPICES FOR FOOD

By now, you've heard that cinnamon lowers blood sugar. Does this mean that you will eat a teaspoon of cinnamon every day and be done with your diabetes? Of course not. But all of the herbs and spices listed starting on page 128 have anti-diabetic and/or anti-inflammatory properties and can be sprinkled

Herbal Use Guidelines

Here are a few guidelines to follow when taking herbs.

1. Most herbs are gentler than conventional drugs, so they also take longer to heal. Take your herbs often and consistently. The therapeutic effects of many herbs only last a few hours in the body, so they need to be taken at least three times a day (unless the bottle says differently).

2. Many herbs should not be taken for longer than 3 weeks—and never for longer than 3 months without the supervision of a trained doctor or herbalist.

3. Being *natural* does not mean that herbs have no side effects. Watch out, and stop immediately if you experience any adverse reaction. Some of the herbs listed in this book have yet to be approved by the FDA, so use caution and discuss your new herbal supplementation with your doctor.

4. In Western medicine, we prescribe medications (and herbs) against a disease: something against high blood pressure, against a cold, against sleeplessness. In traditional Chinese medicine, herbs are given according to the state of the patient: The doctor chooses different herbs in the beginning of a cold, during the worst time of the cold (during the "crisis"), and during recovery from a cold. This means that Chinese practitioners fine-tune the herbs to the patient's condition.

5. The most common unwanted effects of herbs are allergies (you can develop a food allergy to any herb, just as with food) and an upset stomach. The latter is common because the stomach is the port of entry. If the effect is minor and you are not taking the herb for long, you can continue. If it is bothersome, discontinue.

6. Don't take herbs (particularly mushrooms) from the wild if you cannot identify them. About 100 people die from consuming herbs—mostly mushrooms—every year. Contrasted with the thousands of patients who die from using medicinal drugs or from physicians' interventions every year, herbs are pretty safe.

on any meal to help reduce the chronic inflammation in your body. So when you're cooking your next meal, toss in some of the herbs and spices listed below. And don't be afraid to experiment in order to get it just right: By doing this, you'll learn which herbs and spices offer the best flavors for your dishes and how much you prefer to use.

- **Basil** (*Ocimum basilicum*) is that aromatic kitchen herb that reminds us of summer, Italy, and good eating times. It is fragrant in salads, soups, and pesto. In a study of herbal infusions of kitchen herbs, turmeric, rosemary, marjoram, oregano, and basil were the five front-runners in flavonoid content.[28] And basil, specifically, lowers blood sugar.[29]

- **Bilberry** (*Vaccinium myrtillum*) is the European form of blueberries. The berries of this shrub are superior to blueberries because they are blue throughout, whereas our form is blue only on the outside. And the blue color, as you know, carries anthocyanins—the wholesome antioxidants that fight diabetes, strengthen your heart, and lower inflammation and blood fats.[30] A study conducted at the Institute of Public Health and Clinical Nutrition found that regular consumption of fresh bilberries (400 grams daily) reduced inflammation markers and improved glucose tolerance in people with features of metabolic syndrome. When compared with the control group (who maintained their habitual diets), researchers found that the levels of inflammation marker interleukin-6 were 20 percent lower in those who increased their consumption of bilberries.[31] Traditionally, the leaves were used to fight diabetes, but a thorough review of the literature[32] found disappointment only: Stick to the berries, *bil* or *blue*; they also taste better.

- **Bitter melon** (*Momordica charantia*) has anti-diabetic and adaptogenic properties.[33-34] Unfortunately, the name might make people turn away. But give it a try. In a stir-fry with sweet onions and other vegetables, you don't taste the bitterness. It can also be used in a tea or eaten as a vegetable.

- **Black pepper** (*Piper nigrum*) may aid in weight loss and increase the bioavailability of plant compounds in your body.[35] You could call black pepper the synergistic plant: It enhances the actions of other plants (and it is the most-used spice in my kitchen). Black pepper has other advantages as well: Piperine is the ingredient in black pepper that prevents new fat cells from forming.[36]

- **Burdock** (*Arctium lappa*) has anti-diabetic, anti-inflammatory, and antioxidant capacities in its root. It might even protect us from pancreatic cancer,[37] so consider adding this root to your next soup or purchase it in tea bags. It tastes earthy like parsnip.

- **Caraway** (*Carum carvi*) is a forgotten spice because we don't eat much cabbage anymore. Caraway removes some of the unwanted gassiness from cabbage, and the triad of caraway, cabbage, and lamb is a classic for winter stew. Caraway is an anti-diabetic agent and a gentle diuretic.[38] The cabbage itself works against high blood sugar, and grass-fed lamb that grew up outside under the sun is about the best meat you can buy.

- **Cardamom** (*Elettaria cardamomum*) is an Indian herb that aids in weight loss and overall health. Indian spices are known to keep the heart healthy because they function against high lipids and high sugars. They also douse inflammation and prevent cancer from spreading.[39] And cardamom is only one of many Indian spices you can find in local supermarkets. I like to add it to hot beverages, especially in winter.

- **Cayenne and chiles** (*Capsicum annuum*) are in the same family as hot and bell peppers and contain the characteristic ingredient: capsaicin. Like black pepper, capsaicin can aid in weight loss. Hot dishes decrease your appetite, and capsaicin will help to revive your sluggish metabolism,[40] which in turn will shrink your fat stores. Interestingly, if you took the hot pepper in a capsule, it wouldn't have the same effect: The hotness has to hit your stomach lining in order to work.

- **Chamomile** (*Matricaria chamomilla*) lowers blood sugar and prevents diabetic complications by taking the sugar out of your blood and putting it into storage in your liver.[41] And after a day of hard work, there is hardly anything more calming and soothing than a cup of chamomile tea!

- **Chives** (*Allium schoenoprasum*) are in the onion family and are very easy to grow. Indeed, once you have chives in your garden, you usually can't get rid of them—and you shouldn't. They're delicious on scrambled and boiled eggs and in salads, soups, and stews. They have the slight pungency that tells you they must be full of healthy ingredients. Chives are part of what is called the Nordic diet,[42] a nutrition program very much like the one I am proposing here, and one that's definitely more suitable for people with Caucasian background than the standard American diet (SAD). Chives contain vitamins A and C and organosulfur compounds similar to those in garlic, only weaker.[43] That is why chives are used less as a medicine and more as a food. But I found out that using chives in my garden tea enlivens even the blandest leaves. Chives are good for your heart and your circulation and should, therefore, find a place in your diet and your garden.

- **Cinnamon** (*Cinnamomum verum*) lowers blood sugar, according to several studies. But a recent Cochrane meta-analysis did not find significant reductions in fasting blood sugar (FBS), insulin resistance, or hemoglobin A1c.[44] Then again, another meta-analysis found that cinnamon *did* lower hemoglobin A1c.[45] Either way, cinnamon is loaded with phytonutrients that decrease inflammation and may aid in weight loss by lowering cholesterol and speeding up your metabolism. Of course, when you eat cinnamon on a hot bun, you negate its good effects! So try it on beans, lentils, and brown rice, or in meat stews— always without sugar!

- **Cumin** (*Cuminum cyminum*) is a spice in the parsley family that goes well with red lentils or brown rice. Use it generously, as it lowers blood sugar and cholesterol.[46-47] It also has a good effect on the advanced glycation end products (AGEs) that are so damaging in diabetes.

- **Dandelion** (*Taraxacum officinale*) is a wonderful all-around herb, so you should never try to eradicate this "weed" from your garden. This dark, leafy green restocks your body with necessary bitter agents, lowers your blood pressure, and heals your liver.[48] Like nettles, dandelions increase urinary flow and, thereby, support a mild cleansing action. And dandelion is said to help with weight loss,[49] which is paramount for most people with diabetes.

- **Dill** (*Anethum graveolens*) goes well with fish, eggs, or mushrooms. Dill originated in the Middle East and southwestern Russia but had already found its way into European kitchens and apothecaries by the Middle Ages.[50] At that time, it was mainly used to increase milk production in women. Now it is being investigated as an agent against diabetes.[51] James Duke's Ethnobotanical Database lists 70 different chemicals in dill that help fight diabetes.[52]

- **Fennel** (*Foeniculum vulgare*), the vegetable, has a taste like no other—

elegant, with a lingering hint of anise. The seeds, on the other hand, have a stronger aroma; they make the famous fennel tea for colicky babies. Both the vegetable and the seeds contain chemicals that work against diabetes.[53] Anethole, one of the phytochemicals found in fennel, blocks several inflammatory agents in the body and fights cancer.[54] Indians chew on fennel seeds after a meal to clean their teeth and freshen their breath. If you like the flavor of strong cough drops, fennel is a good cough suppressant (in addition to helping with diabetes and gastrointestinal ailments), and the essential oil is available in capsules.

• **Fenugreek** (*Trigonella foenum-graecum*) has a strong taste. You might want to use it anyway, though, because a study performed at the Jaipur Diabetes and Research Center showed that regular consumption of fenugreek decreased insulin resistance and improved glycemic control in people with type 2 diabetes.[55] It is a spice that works best in soups and stews.

• **Garlic** (*Allium sativum*) gives Italian and Mediterranean cuisines their specific flavors, together with basil, oregano, and olive oil. Garlic is good for your heart and protects you from cancer,[56] as do onions, shallots, and chives, which are in the same plant family. Garlic exhibits the strongest anti-inflammatory[57] force among them, suppressing exactly those cytokines acting up in diabetes. But garlic can do more: It lowers blood sugars and lipids, as well as C-reactive protein—a marker of inflammation.[58] Pretty much any vegetable becomes palatable when dressed with garlic and olive oil. In a pinch, I use dried garlic in my kitchen, well aware that it does not have the same good effects as fresh; raw, freshly sliced garlic seems to have the maximal potency.[59]

• **Ginger** (*Zingiber officinale*) is the perfect herb to fight diabetes and high blood lipids because it attacks diabetes from several sides, and even helps with weight loss.[60] In fact, a 2012 study conducted by nutritionists at Columbia University found that subjects burned an extra 43 calories after consuming a breakfast that contained a hot ginger beverage. In addition, those who drank the beverage, which contained 2 grams of dry ginger powder, reported greater satiety 3 hours later than those who didn't consume the ginger.[61] And in a separate study published in *Plant Foods for Human Nutrition*, diabetic patients who consumed 3 grams of dry ginger powder in divided doses for 30 days experienced a significant reduction in blood glucose (17%), triglyceride (9%), total cholesterol (8%), LDL (12%), and VLDL cholesterol (9%).[62] Most of the time, I have fresh ginger at home and cut a few thin slices into my hot tea. Taken early on, ginger nips a cold in the bud. And a study shows that AGEs are basically thrown out by ginger and have no chance to settle in tissue. In one study, ginger stopped the AGEs from building up in the lens of the eye, preventing cataracts.[63] Use this Asian spice in as many dishes as you can. It goes well with meat and poultry dishes, and vegetarian fare, too.

- **Ginkgo biloba** is an ancient tree—one of the earliest trees that appeared on Earth. Its leaves enhance bloodflow to most organs and are, therefore, used against dementia and arterial diseases, including Raynaud's.[64-65] And, for our purposes, it limits diabetic damage by reducing oxidative stress and inflammation in the cells.

- **Gymnema sylvestre** contains phytocompounds called *gymnemic acids*, which work against diabetes and obesity.[66] It is the tea I most often recommend to patients with diabetes. Its bitter taste resets your taste buds after you've eaten something sugary, and it seems to relieve the sugar cravings that would follow otherwise.

- **Herbes de Provence** is a new-fangled invention with little Provençale verity to it. What you can buy now in stores is practical, but expensive. Nevertheless, it goes well with mushrooms, roasted potatoes, and ground beef. And the individual herbs—thyme, rosemary, savory, fennel, basil, and lavender—included in herbes de Provence have all been shown to have antioxidant potency against inflammation.

- **Horsetail** (*Equisetum arvense*) is sometimes recommended for diabetics, but I would be careful, as it is also a bit harsh on the kidneys, especially when taken for longer than a few days. Since horsetail is also a potent diuretic, it is mainly used to cleanse the diabetic body of toxins, but it can also make your potassium levels dip too low. It is contraindicated for people with kidney disease, and the beginnings of that might be present in early diabetics. So only use this herb under the advice of a physician or experienced herbalist.

- **Huckleberry** is a general term for plants in the *Vaccinium* and *Gaylussacia* genera. They show similar actions against diabetes and metabolic syndrome as bilberries and blueberries.

- **Italian seasoning** is less expensive than herbes de Provence but give a similarly nice flavor to otherwise bland dishes. Again, there are different mixtures, but the main ingredients are oregano, thyme, basil, parsley, and sage. Some mixtures also contain black pepper and bay leaves. All contain inflammation-opposing antioxidants helpful in the fight against diabetes.

- **Linden flowers** (*Tilia* spp.) contain flavonoids that are potent antioxidants. Most often they are used to treat colds and coughs, but the fragrant tea also helps against diabetes.

- **Marjoram** (*Origanum majorana*) is another one of those miracle herbs that stop AGEs from harming your cells. It is often used on roasted chicken or other poultry, or in poultry stuffing—probably to counteract the damage roasting can do. I like to make my stuffing with apples, chestnuts or nuts, and a handful of dried marjoram—without bread crumbs. If you find the herb fresh, consider yourself lucky and put it on beans, salads, and soups.

- **Motherwort** (*Leonurus cardiaca*) is good for your heart. While it has no proven direct effect on diabetes, a diabetic heart is always in danger, so it is good to use this herb. It also contains nutrients that fight cancer.

- **Mustard seed** comes from two genera: *Brassica* and *Sinapis*. They both help with weight loss, and mustard greens are wonderful with olive oil and garlic.

- **Neem** (*Azadirachta indica*) not only has great antibacterial oil in its seeds that can be used on wounds, scrapes, and burns, but it can also be used as a tea and has strong anti-diabetic effects. Neem tea should not be used internally by children and pregnant women because it can damage the liver.

- **Parsley** (*Petroselinum* spp.) has great anti-inflammatory action. I like it on sautéed carrots with a dab of ghee and white pepper. Most people don't know that in larger amounts, parsley is dangerous for pregnant women. Otherwise, it strengthens the immune system.

- **Peppermint** (*Mentha* x *piperita*) contains natural antioxidants that fight diabetes, heart disease, aging, and cancer.[67] And it adds great flavor to teas. Try to get it loose and fresh instead of in tea bags. Peppermint relaxes the muscles that close the stomach from the esophagus; people with reflux should, therefore, avoid peppermint. For all others it is a tasty tea that aids digestion.

- **Rooibos** (*Aspalathus linearis*) is a South African bush, and its leaves burst with antioxidants. The dark brown tea brewed from this bush looks like any black tea, but doesn't contain caffeine, making it a perfect bedtime tea. And wouldn't you know it—it is full of polyphenols that work against diabetes.[68]

- **Rosemary** (*Rosmarinus officinalis*) is a heart tonic, important in the treatment of metabolic syndrome. Rosemary's most active phytochemical, *carnosol*, lowers oxidative stress, and this is effective in fighting inflammation and cancer.[69] You can harvest these properties by using rosemary in your cooking, especially when you're preparing meats, stews, and stir-fries. Or try brewing a relaxing rosemary tea.

- **Sage** (*Salvia officinalis*) contains antioxidants that have been shown to fight diabetes.[70] Its strong taste works well in stews, while the tea is soothing and calming. Like all aromatic kitchen herbs, sage is high in polyphenols; its rosmarinic acid content is higher than in rosemary itself.[71] That phenolic compound shows promise in the battle against Alzheimer's.[72] Sage and honey tea works against viral and bacterial colds because when sage and honey are combined, they have enhanced anti-germ power.

- **Savory** comes in two genera: summer savory (*Satureja hortensis*) and winter savory (*S. montana*). In Germany, both are called *bean herbs* and are used on green beans and lima beans, and any other bean you can imagine. Both of these savories have a high antioxidant capacity.[73]

- **Stevia** (*Stevia rebaudiana*) is the only sweetener that is not detrimental to those with diabetes—even though it is many times sweeter than table sugar. While using stevia won't help to eliminate your sweet tooth, stevia does have positive effects on postprandial blood sugar and insulin levels.[74] You can grow the plant in a pot on your windowsill. One little leaf goes a long way.

- **Tarragon** (*Artemisia dracunculus*) is a fine herb that has been shown to lower insulin resistance and decrease overeating in diabetics.[75] The French kind (var. sativa) does not easily propagate, but the Russian and American kinds (*A. dracunculus*) have spread invariably over most of the temperate world. Unfortunately, the American species does not have the same hypoglycemic effect, so you might have to shell out a bit more for the French type.

- **Thyme** (*Thymus* spp.) contains 75 active phytochemicals that work against diabetes, and its delicious aroma enhances any dish. It supports inflammation-fighting cytokines and helps certain immune cells (macrophages) secrete agents that douse inflammation.[76]

- **Turmeric** (*Curcuma longa*), the yellow root popular in Indian cuisine and always present in curries, is probably the best herb or spice for preventing cancer. It is an ideal spice for those with diabetes, as research has proven it has anti-inflammatory, anti-aging, antioxidant, neuroprotective, anti-atherosclerotic, heart-protecting, weight reducing, and anti-infectious actions.[77] All of these benefits have been attributed to its main ingredient, *curcumin*.[78]

  According to a study published in the journal *Diabetes Care*, 240 people, all of whom had been diagnosed with prediabetes, were assigned to take either daily curcumin capsules (1500 mg) or a placebo for 9 months. At the end of the study, researchers found that 16.4 percent of subjects who took the placebo developed type 2 diabetes, while no one who took the daily dose of curcumin developed diabetes.[79]

- **White (Chinese) chrysanthemum flowers** (*C. indicum*) make a fragrant tea that is popular in China. You should use it at the beginning of a cold and to clear your liver and eyes. It's important to know that it has been used successfully to fight obesity.[80]

As you can see, there are a variety of anti-diabetic herbs available to you. So whether you choose to incorporate your herbs as a tonic, add them to your new nutritious meals, or drink them in teas, you can be assured that you're getting all of the health benefits and anti-inflammatory actions you need to begin your journey toward health. And if you're itching to get into the kitchen to use some of the herbs we've discussed in this chapter, skip ahead to Chapter 14, where you'll find easy, delicious recipes that show you how to make use of the healing phytonutrients in herbs.

Movement

9

....

Those who think they have no time for exercise
will sooner or later have to find time for illness.

—EDWARD STANLEY (1779–1849)

Exercise—Oh, *No!*

Most people don't like to exercise, so they don't—even if they have heard
that it will benefit their health. If you are one of these people, you're in luck
because I'm going to teach you how to enjoy physical activity. Why? Well,
research provides ample evidence that movement lowers inflammation in
your body. And contrary to popular belief, you don't have to make the gym
your second home in order to reap the benefits of activity. Newer research
has shown that even small amounts of activity can improve metabolic health
and even reduce your risk of developing type 2 diabetes. All you have to do
is add a little *movement* here and there throughout your day. In fact, a 2012
study in the *European Journal of Applied Physiology*, 29 healthy, but sedentary
men and women were assigned to either a reduced-exertion high-intensity
interval training intervention or to a control group. While those in the control group maintained their sedentary lifestyle, subjects in the training group
completed 10-minute exercise sessions 3 days a week for 6 weeks. The exercise sessions consisted of mostly low-intensity cycling with brief 10- to
20-second sprints. At the end of the 6-week period, insulin sensitivity had

significantly increased by 28 percent in the male training group, despite low ratings of exertion. And both the men and women had increased their aerobic capacity by 15 percent and 12 percent, respectively.[1]

I favor staying active all day with little chores or movements over going to a gym. Why? Too much repetitive exercise increases your risk of developing injuries, while steadily moving throughout your day does not. And since both make your body use up more energy, both will help you lose weight. The one advantage a hard workout has is that you sweat out toxins, but heat exposure can accomplish the same thing.

You may believe that athletes, as a group, are healthier, but they're not: They are just fitter, meaning their muscles are stronger. But they may die prematurely from heart disease and suffer from worn-out organs and joints as a result of excessive exercise.[2] And since athletes sometimes consume foods (like protein powders that can overburden their kidneys) and substances (like steroids) in huge quantities, their health tends to suffer as a result. For the average person, incorporating small amounts of movement into each day will result in decreased inflammation and a marked improvement in overall health.

Exercise and Inflammation

So how does exercise reduce inflammation? The answer is complicated, as exercise works on so many levels. Basically, exercise increases short-term inflammation and reduces long-term inflammation.[3] When your muscles ache after a workout, acute inflammation is taking place in your body. But if you exercise daily, you will reap the benefits: reduced glycated hemoglobin A1c, increased insulin sensitivity, increased oxygen consumption, and reduced chronic inflammation. Interestingly, studies show that remaining sedentary and training very hard *both* increase oxidative stress on cells—one of the markers of inflammation—which drives the generation of type 2 diabetes.[4-5]

Sebastian Kneipp put it like this: *"Too little* weakens, *just right* strengthens, *too much* hurts."* The scientific name for this concept is *hormesis*: a small stimulus that sets something in motion for the better, when a large stimulus would kill the organism.[6] A good example of this is the difference between *endurance exercise* and *resistance exercise*. In endurance exercise, you have high repetition of contractile activity, but low resistance. In resistance exercise, you

Rita's Story

Rita was recently retired. For 40 years, she had successfully sold jewelry and considered herself a cut above other salespersons. Within a few months of retiring, she'd gained 20 pounds. Her older sister had passed away from diabetes and Parkinson's, and Rita worried that with her weight gain, she would suffer the same fate. And it didn't help matters that she disliked cooking. She and her husband often resorted to eating takeout or processed food from a box. For "health," she would sometimes throw in a salad.

My assessment was that dairy was Rita's worst enemy. Luckily, she did not like sweets at all—but her husband did. When I tried to explain that dairy was inflammatory and addictive—and linked to Parkinson's and diabetes—she listened, but she didn't seem convinced. Even calculating her BMI at nearly 30 did not convince her. I also encouraged her to be more physically active by going for a daily walk. She frowned and declared that she had begun to do a little gardening since her retirement, and that should suffice.

It was only when her A1c came back as 6.4 and she received the diagnosis of type 2 diabetes that she became motivated to walk for a few minutes every day and focus on eliminating dairy products from her diet. She slowly lost 15 pounds and her A1c dropped to 6.1, where it stalled. Frustrated, Rita claimed she could not lose any more weight and her A1c couldn't get any lower. But then she noticed that her husband had begun walking. He even bought himself a pedometer to count his steps, and he slowly built up his endurance to 3 to 5 miles per day. And his commitment motivated her.

Rita also noticed that her long-standing nasal congestion had vanished just from making those few minor changes to her lifestyle. These observations renewed her drive: Soon, Rita had a group of women who walked with her every day. She was now also convinced that dairy had been bad for her all her life, and she spread the word among her friends. Encouraged by her progress, Rita learned to cook and began to add anti-inflammatory foods into her diet. And over the next few months, her A1c came down to 5.6 and she lost the rest of her retirement weight gain.

Rita was so thrilled her diabetes had vanished that she maintained her new lifestyle and even became an advocate for nondairy diets. In the years that followed, Rita lost another 5 pounds, for a total of a 25-pound weight loss.

have low repetition, but high resistance. People often combine those two principles by using weights and fast movements to get added benefits (and sometimes receive added pain). But I am not interested in building muscles; I am interested in getting you off of the couch the easy way.

Why Don't We Exercise More?

Disclosure: Nobody ever wanted me on their sports team. I was always the least-athletic girl in class. I could not throw a ball and was deathly afraid of being hit by one in dodgeball. I learned to swim well enough to keep my head above water, but could not swim fast. I also couldn't run fast. I couldn't even hit a baseball. The only physical activity I volunteered for was rowing a boat in the old canals of Hamburg. I would park the boat under the lovely green curtain of a weeping willow and read a book for hours before rowing home.

At the age of 12, I caught tuberculosis and spent a year in the hospital. Afterward, I was always exempted from participating in school sports. I hated sports, and thought I was done with them for life—and I didn't mind. Then, around the age of 30, I began to feel stiff. I began to practice yoga because as a medical student, I knew that not moving could be deadly.

Many people experience a similar inability to perform or disinterest in participating in athletic endeavors. And physicians have not been much help by encouraging people to put in at least three sessions of one and a half hours per week of aerobic exercise. Have we heeded their advice? No. But is it because we are stubborn and willful, or are there reasons behind our resistance?

Less Is More

Nothing is more discouraging than being told that only extreme cardiovascular training will keep you healthy. Upon hearing this, people tend to immediately give up hope of incorporating activity into their lives because even the thought of going to the gym is too much to handle. After all, we live in the real world and have families, a job (or two), and numerous daily responsibilities, so we just don't have that much time to devote to anything else. But here's some good news: Since research is finding that extreme exercise might be doing more harm than good by increasing the markers for inflammation, we need to focus on small, quick movements. And these quick movements will be easy to complete and incorporate into your daily life.

I stopped believing a long time ago that people have to exercise hard to see results; I noticed that my patients showed marked improvements after completing even small amounts of daily movement. And the Centenarian Study has shown that people who live to a ripe old age didn't spend much time exercising.[7] Instead, they spend time with friends, putter around their house and garden, and live for a worthwhile cause. I am not saying that you should stop exercising, especially if you enjoy it. But like everything, you should do it in moderation—a minute here and there every day. And because we're focusing on reducing inflammation, these movements will give you better health than hitting the gym three times a week.

Your Movement Progress

Any movement you do will immediately register with your metabolism. With every little step or activity, you are improving your diabetes. You may begin to notice that you're feeling better within a day or two after you start incorporating daily movement. But it could take longer, depending on the amount of inflammation you have and the current state of your diabetes. The

The Benefits of Outdoor Activity

A meta-analysis revealed that being active outdoors is more beneficial than remaining indoors.[8] Researchers tried to figure out if there are benefits to exercise in a natural outdoor environment versus a confined gym. They found that participants often reported that they had more energy, less tension, and generally better moods when they exercised in a natural outdoor environment. And when compared to those who completed indoor activity, these participants also said they received greater satisfaction upon completing the outdoor activities—and were more likely to do them again in the future.

important thing to remember is that the moment you begin to move with purpose, you have begun to change your body and heal your inflamed metabolism. From there, you can gradually increase your amount of daily activity and create a routine that works for you.

Movement for Beginners

Think back to when you were a child. Was there a specific activity that you enjoyed? The idea here is to recapture the joy you experienced during activities at that time in your life. By associating your daily movements with a positive memory, you'll be more likely to stick with them, which is important for beginners. If you can't think of a specific activity from childhood, take a look at the movements listed in this chapter; they're quick, easy, and designed to fight the diabetes-causing inflammation in your body.

Water Movement

If you are overweight or have been diagnosed with diabetes and your weight bogs down your joints, the best movement you can do is in water. Intuitively, it feels like exercising in the water is easier. But a recent study has shown that you get the same benefits from water exercise as from land exercise, without the joint strain you might experience on land.[9] While it's best to do your water movements in an ocean, river, or lake to avoid chemicals, a nonchlorinated pool is also acceptable. Because water movement is less damaging to joints and muscles, it works well not only for those who are overweight, but also for people who have an injury, arthritis, or brittle bones. See Chapter 11 for more tips on how water can heal your body.

Daily Walks

Try to walk for 10 minutes every day—rain or shine. It's important to get outside as much as possible, but if you find that the ground is icy from winter weather conditions, you can open some windows and walk around inside until you're able to get outdoors again. And because you're just starting out, don't push yourself too hard and stay at a steady pace.

During your walks, your muscles burn sugar and fat, and this is how your metabolism heals, ultimately helping to rid your body of chronic inflammation. So don't focus on trying to lose weight when you walk, because this will happen automatically. Instead, focus on all of the health benefits you're receiving from your walks and take in the beauty around you.

- **Memory improvement.** A recent study showed that brisk walks boost memory in older adults.[10] When subjects walked 6 to 9 miles during the week, they had better brain function. Interestingly, additional walking didn't seem to have any greater effect on the brain. So what does this mean for you? Think of it this way: If you walk 10 minutes in one direction and then turn around and walk back to your initial starting point during lunch each day, not only are you fighting that inflammation in your body, but you're also improving your memory— and this makes for a more productive afternoon.

- **Lower blood pressure and reduced risk of disease.** Research has shown that the benefits of walking are even greater if you walk on uneven surfaces, like on pebbles, at a beach, or on hilly terrain.[11] Walking on pebbles lowers high blood pressure and even decreases your chance of developing Parkinson's disease. That's because when you walk on uneven surfaces you use more muscles and consequently more brain cells.

- **Increased vitamin D.** When you walk outdoors, exposure to natural light increases the vitamin D production under your skin. Vitamin D has become an important research focus, as it wards off bone loss, multiple sclerosis, cancer, and infections. And since people with type 2 diabetes can be prone to developing infections, this is especially helpful in the fight against diabetes.

The Five Tibetan Rites

Studies show that moving your muscles reduces the disorderly diabetic state of affairs in your body. But does this mean you have to get a gym membership or spend your weekends jogging? No. Prehistoric men and women did not jog. They *roamed* all day, more or less. On average, men roamed for 7 hours, namely while hunting, while women spent about 4 hours roaming, namely while gathering—and then did housework. And since we have the same ancient bodies as our ancestors, we need to get back to our primal way of leisurely movement.

Our ancestors were constantly moving and would only run when there was danger. Otherwise, they took it slow and easy, performing varied movements throughout the day. So don't think of your daily activity as a "routine." Instead, think of it as a variety of movement. No single activity or movement uses all of your muscles. So whether you choose to walk, do yoga, or simply perform some light jumping jacks, variety is the key. But since we have so little time in our modern society, these varied movements need to be simple, short, and effective.

My preferred activities have evolved throughout the years, but one thing has remained constant: Every movement has been based on the Five Tibetan Rites. According to Peter Kelder, who first published a booklet about this series of movements, the Five Tibetan Rites were allegedly unearthed by a British officer desperate to regain his youth. These yogalike movements were designed to create a continuous stream of motion consisting of five exercises, each with 21 repetitions (based on the Tibetan belief that this is a perfect number). But even though 21 repetitions is ideal, you should start out with only 1 or 2 reps if you're just beginning to incorporate new movements into your daily life. And never, ever, do more than 21 reps of each movement in a single day.

Repeating a movement 21 times will usually take about a minute or less. And, believe it or not, completing five or six of those little exercises will make a huge difference in your life. By doing 21 repetitions of any movement, you're giving your muscles a workout and building strength and new muscles, while minimizing your risk of injury. The point is not to bulk you up, but to make your muscles responsive to insulin again and functioning in a way that will leave you glowing with health. Slowly but surely, you will crave more physical activity once you see the results.

You should always begin slowly and mindfully. Later, you can do your 21 repetitions faster, according to how you feel, because your body's requirements are unique: Some people need to be driven harder, while some prefer to move gently.

So what are the Five Tibetan Rites? For easier learning, I started the names of all the Rites with an S.

1. **Spinning.** *How to do it:* Stand straight with your arms outstretched at shoulder height. Begin slowly spinning in clockwise circles. Try to complete 21 spins, but stop if you become dizzy. When you've finished

spinning, give yourself a few moments to make sure any dizziness is gone. *Why you should do it:* Spinning revives your metabolism and prepares your body for weight loss.

2. **Straightening.** *How to do it:* Lie on your back with your hands by your sides. Lift your feet straight up until your legs are perpendicular to the floor and your soles face the ceiling, then lower them slowly. Lift 21 times total, or until you cannot keep your back pressed into the floor any longer. Make sure to rest between lifts. And if you experience any pain, bend your knees when lifting and lowering your legs. This will relieve any tension in your lower back. *Why you should do it:* Straightening builds abdominal strength, therefore, targeting inflammatory belly fat.

3. **Swaying.** *How to do it:* Kneel on the floor with your hands at the sides of your legs. Curl in your toes and lower your head while slowly bending forward. Next, lift your head back up and bend backward as much as possible. Do this 21 times, or until you are tired. *Note:* If you don't have a strong core, use extra caution when performing this movement. Try to complete the movement without bending backward. *Why you should do it:* Swaying strengthens your entire back, making it more flexible by separating each spinal vertebra from the others.

4. **Sitting.** *How to do it:* Sit on the floor with your legs outstretched. Place your hands flat on the ground next to your sides with your fingers together and pointing slightly outward. Push your weight into your feet as you lift your middle section, so that your belly forms a table: Your arms and calves are perpendicular to the floor while your thighs and torso are horizontal. Let your head fall loosely backward. Do this 21 times, or until you feel tired. *Note:* This movement can be especially difficult for some people due to the strain it can put on your wrists. If you find that it hurts you to complete this movement, skip it. *Why you should do it:* Sitting strengthens your back, abdominal muscles, arms, shoulders, and legs—almost every single muscle in your body.

5. **Swinging.** *How to do it:* From a standing position, lower your hands to the floor, creating an upside-down V with your body (also known as a Downward Dog yoga pose). Next, tuck your chin into your chest and lower your hips down toward the floor (as if you are at the top of a pushup). Swing 21 times between these two poses, or until you grow tired. *Why you should do it:* It strengthens your arms, legs, and back.

Note: This is also one of the hardest movements if you are not already in the habit of doing pushups, so take your time and only move as much as your body allows.

Even though they are still referred to as the Five Tibetan Rites, a sixth Rite was added:

6. **Swirling.** *How to do it:* This is a popular yoga exercise that swirls your stomach around with extremely deep breathing. Begin by inhaling deeply and then exhaling forcefully as you lean over and rest your hands on your thighs. Without taking in another breath, suck your stomach in and up as much as you can before pushing it back out again. Do this 21 times. As your stomach muscles develop, you can begin pushing out your left abdominal muscles and then your right abdominal muscles, which is known as swirling. *Why you should do it:* Swirling is good for your stomach because it fights belly fat. It also facilitates bowel movements.

Beyond the Rites

Many patients who've tried the Five Tibetan Rites have returned to tell me that they enjoy the movements and are still doing them daily. But it's important to remember that every body is different, so pay attention to your body's needs—and stop if any movement begins to hurt. After all, the Five Tibetan Rites are a little tough, especially in the beginning. So I've developed some simpler 1-minute alternatives to ease you into the joy of experiencing activity again.

You'll notice that, like the Five Tibetan Rites, these alternatives call for 21 reps because this gives you enough movement but doesn't put undue stress on your muscles and joints. And remember: You should only complete one set of each movement every day, to avoid injury.

If the Five Tibetan Rites work for you, by all means, stay with them! But if you find that you're struggling or experiencing any pain, take a look at the 1-minute movements for some simple, quick alternatives.

1-MINUTE MOVEMENTS

Did you know research has shown that sitting is directly linked to the development of type 2 diabetes and obesity?[12] According to a 2009 study published in the journal *Diabetes*, the amount of time people without diabetes spent sedentary predicted higher levels of fasting insulin, regardless of the amount of time they spent doing moderate- and vigorous-intensity activity.[13] In fact, chairs and sofas are later developments and provide none of the benefits our ancestors received from their "seating method": squatting. Squatting aids in digestion, strengthens leg and pelvic muscles, and even reduces abdominal fat.[14] Sitting all day sends signals to your cells that they are not needed. This is why it's important to incorporate daily movement into your life and break up the time you spend seated.

As a writer, I like a concept that can easily be implemented during short work breaks. So in addition to the Five Tibetan Rites, here are some easy 1-minute movements that can be easily slipped into your busy day—anytime, anywhere.

- **Get down on the ground.** *How to do it:* For a child, this is the easiest thing in the world. But as we age, we find that this becomes harder and harder. If you don't do any other movements in this chapter, this is the *one thing* you need to do every single day: Sit down on the ground and get back up again. *Why you should do it:* If you don't sit down on the ground, sooner or later, you won't be able to lower yourself down to that level. Many people who fondly recall crouching under the big family table as a child or romping around in the living room with the dog can't get down on the ground anymore, much to their surprise. And if they do, the odds are that they won't be able to get back up again because their arms and legs aren't strong enough to push them back up again. In fact, a Brazilian study has shown a direct correlation between how much help you need to sit and rise from the floor and your risk of mortality: Those who required more assistance had a higher mortality rate than those who could rise from the floor on their own.[15]

  So this is your homework today: Get down on the floor, and get back up again. If you require assistance the first few times, make sure someone is around to help you. By doing this once every day, you will strengthen the muscles you use for walking and balance. And if you fall in the future, you will have the strength to pull yourself back up.

- **Standing balance.** *How to do it:* Anytime you're standing still (while brushing your teeth, waiting for the bus, or talking on the phone), stand on one leg. After about 30 seconds, switch legs. If you have good balance, try moving your lifted leg from side to side or back and forth. *Why you should do it:* This is easily the exercise that gives you the most bang for your buck, so to speak. Not only does it strengthen your leg and pelvic muscles, but it also improves your balance and coordination, ultimately reducing your risk of falls. Standing on one leg also increases bone mass in your legs and spine, counteracting osteopenia and osteoporosis, and thus preventing those nasty hip fractures.

- **Walking side step.** *How to do it:* Begin by extending your right foot to the side. Next, cross your left foot over your right foot. Do this 21 times, moving to the right, and then repeat beginning with your left foot, returning to your starting position. *Why you should do it:* This works entirely different muscles than you normally use when walking. It also uses your brain differently, which has been shown to help fight dementia.

- **Bed board.** *How to do it:* While lying on your back in bed, dig your heels and the lower part of the back of your head into the mattress. Next, press your chin into your chest and arch your back. Breathe in and out before relaxing again. Do this 21 times. *Why you should do it:* This move strengthens all of your back muscles, especially your upper back and neck. It also tones the flesh around your hips and works like a charm against a double chin.

- **Tongue stretch.** *How to do it:* After you finish brushing your teeth every morning and night, stick out your tongue as far as you can 21 times. *Why you should do it:* The tongue stretch works your platysma—the flat muscle that might sag under your chin—and helps to prevent or eliminate a double chin. This movement is so beneficial that you may repeat it as often as you desire.

- **Swimming on dry land.** *How to do it:* Lie facedown on the floor. Lift your arms and legs slightly above the ground and imitate swimming the breast stroke. Do this 21 times. *Why you should do it:* This movement strengthens your back muscles and actually helps to relieve constipation. It also makes you get down on the floor and then back up again, which slows aging and keeps your hips nimble.

- **Jumps.** *How to do it:* On the spot, jump up and down 21 times. *Note:* Use caution if you have ankle, knee, or hip problems. *Why you should do it:* Jumping up and down exercises your legs and spine. This is the quickest of these movements and can be done when you're waiting for something or someone.

- **Shoulder squeeze.** *How to do it:* Try to push your shoulder blades together and hold for a few seconds. Do this 21 times. *Why you should do it:* This move helps to improve posture and loosen the muscles of your upper back.

- **Rocking.** *How to do it:* Sit on the floor with your chin tucked down into your chest, and hug your knees close to your torso. Slowly roll back onto your curved spine and rock back up again. Do this 21 times. *Why you should do it:* This movement works your abdominals and helps to keep your spine flexible. And by getting you down on the floor, it works your hips and legs when you get back up.

- **Arm extensions.** *How to do it:* Grab some light dumbbells or a heavy book. Keeping your arms straight, lift the object out and bring it up over your head. Then lower the object down behind your head before raising it back up over your head again. Lower your arms back down to your waist. Do this 21 times. *Why you should do it:* This movement works your triceps and prevents or eliminates arm flab. It also strengthens the muscles of your upper back, shoulders, and arms.

Get Moving

Because research has shown that extreme exercise can actually worsen the inflammation in your body, it's important to begin slowly. Start by strolling around your neighborhood and doing one or two different movements each day. This is all you need to do to begin eliminating the chronic inflammation inside your body. Gradually add a new movement until you're completing five or six movements each day—and make sure you mix them up!

- **Backward bend.** *How to do it:* Lying faceup on a balance ball, roll your upper back over the ball. Each time you roll backward, lift your arms over your head, and lower them back down as you roll forward again. (If you don't have a balance ball, you can also do this movement by hanging backward off the edge of your bed.) Do this 21 times. *Why you should do it:* Bending works on your upper back and improves your posture without putting undue strain on your lower back.

- **Grounding.** *How to do it:* These are basically knee bends, but I call this movement *grounding* because it strengthens your legs—and if you think about grounding instead of bending, you do them better. Stand with both feet together and knees slightly bent. Squat down slowly, and then rise up again. Repeat 21 times. In the beginning, try holding onto a chair for extra support. Once you feel comfortable, you can perform this movement without support. *Note:* If you have trouble with this movement, only do it 5 times, and bend down only as far as you can comfortably go. *Why you should do it:* Grounding strengthens your leg muscles and improves your balance. It also improves your posture without putting undue strain on your lower back.

- **Hanging.** *How to do it:* Hanging is just another word for pullups. If you have access to a pullup bar, begin by grabbing the bar with your palms facing in. Now it might seem impossible to complete even one pullup, let alone 21, so don't be afraid to rest between each pullup to avoid injury. If you don't have access to a pullup bar, try bending forward and resting your hands on a table while pulling your body slightly down and back (without bending your knees). *Why you should do it:* Hanging will lengthen your spine and strengthen your arms.

- **Reaching.** *How to do it:* This is the movement that I enjoy the most. In one hand, hold a heavy ball (I use a 6-pound ball at home), a large book, or a filled water bottle, and reach up as high as you can. (You'll feel your whole side stretching.) Do this 21 times, and then repeat with the other arm. *Note:* Be sure to only work one side at a time. If you reached with both hands at the same time, you wouldn't get the same effect. *Why you should do it:* Reaching slims your waist, strengthens your arms, and melts away arm flab.

- **Swinging back and forth.** *How to do it:* Take a heavy ball or book and move it back and forth from one hand to the other in a smooth swinging motion 21 times. *Why you should do it:* Swinging strengthens your back and tones your arms.

These movements work because they make you practice mindfulness throughout the day: You stand on one leg while waiting for the bus. You get up from the computer and squeeze your shoulder blades. You are in the bathroom and stick out your tongue a few extra times. This program keeps you aware of your body and the fact that it needs attention and pampering.

Weekend Movements

The beginner movements are perfect to get you through your busy week, but if you want more variety or a greater challenge, consider doing some extra

No Time for Exercise?

Is your schedule so hectic that your days pass by without any movement at all? Perhaps you're chained to your desk trying to meet a deadline. Or maybe you have an illness that makes completing ordinary tasks feel like an extreme challenge. If this sounds familiar, here's the ideal exercise for you: micromovements!

Lie on your back—in bed, on the floor—and pull back one shoulder. Release, and pull back the other shoulder. Do this 21 times for optimal benefits. Done repeatedly, it releases muscle contractions and loosens your back by moving your spine. While it may seem like it's not doing much, micromovements are like a mini yoga session and will give you most of the benefits of exercise: suppleness, body awareness, improved posture, and muscle relaxation.

Once you get the hang of it, you can do micromovements every-where—especially when you are waiting around or bored. Why not use that time for a little rejuvenation? If you find that you're really limited in what you can do within a specific time or space, think about purchasing a balance cushion online or in a local store. These cushions are relatively inexpensive and create a form of unconscious micromovement by mak-ing you constantly adjust your sitting stability. But if you're not as limited with your time, don't be afraid to get creative: Use your surroundings to come up with your own micromovements to give yourself a little variety!

activity on the weekends. You may find that you get motivation from joining a class or signing up for a bigger adventure. Here are some ideas, in order of least taxing to most strenuous.

- **Tai chi.** This ancient practice (also called shadow boxing) is a Chinese martial art. It is based on completing gentle, flowing, artful movements. *Why you should do it:* Tai chi tones the whole body, improves balance (which prevents falls), and strengthens concentration.

- **Yoga.** The moment you enroll in a yoga class, you have already proven that your body can influence your mind—and any great learning can happen from there. Originally from India, yoga combines gentle, calming movements with steady breathing techniques to reduce stress. *Why you should do it:* Newer research is showing that yoga has numerous health benefits—most importantly, reducing inflammation.[16]

- **Gardening.** Growing flowers for beauty or herbs and vegetables for food and health will help you reconnect with the Earth. Having a garden makes you move constantly, even if it's just a small strip on your windowsill. *Why you should do it:* Not only will keeping a garden help you get back to basics, but you'll also meet your daily movement goals while working on a new hobby. It's really one of the only movements that incorporates all of The Five Health Essentials.

- **Biking.** Riding a bicycle is the perfect transportation for short distances. If your current health condition doesn't allow you to do this and you have access to a stationary bike, try to use it! While you won't get the benefit of fresh air, a modern stationary bike will help you keep track of your heart rate, breathing, and distance. *Why you should do it:* Biking not only improves your health by getting you to move more, it also provides your body with vitamin D through exposure to the sun. You'll also gain muscle mass and lower your blood sugar with every minute you spend on your bicycle.

- **Skiing.** Once you begin to regain energy and excel at the movements in this chapter, you may desire a bigger challenge. (And at this point, you've likely built up the strength to take on a new, more demanding activity.) *Why you should do it:* Skiing is the perfect sport when not much else will lure you outside during the cold winter months. And you don't even have to go to a pricey resort or lodge: You can cross-country ski right outside your door when the snow piles up. And don't be intimidated if you haven't skied before: This sport can be done—

Zen Running

I am not a big fan of jogging or running: It typically causes too many injuries. But if you feel that you need to go for a light jog, this gentle Zen running can be done by almost everyone. (Make sure to consult with your doctor if your diabetes or weight is of concern.) When you're running, try to be as graceful and gentle as possible, and don't run more than 3 days a week.

Alternate running and walking according to the schedule below—and don't run on 2 consecutive days so that your body has a chance to heal after each run. Make sure to take your time and run slowly. *Hint:* Always run with your mouth closed, breathing through your nose. If you find that you have to breathe through your mouth, slow down and take lighter steps.

Your Zen Running Schedule

- **Week 1:** 2-minute run, 1-minute walk. Repeat 10 times.
- **Week 2:** 3-minute run, 1-minute walk. Repeat 9 times.
- **Week 3:** 4-minute run, 1-minute walk. Repeat 7 times.
- **Week 4:** 5-minute run, 1-minute walk. Repeat 5 times.
- **Week 5:** 7-minute run, 1-minute walk. Repeat 4 times.
- **Week 6:** 9-minute run, 1-minute walk. Repeat 3 times.
- **Week 7:** 10-minute run, 1-minute walk. Repeat 3 times.
- **Week 8:** 15-minute run, 1-minute walk. Repeat 2 times.
- **Week 9:** 30-minute run

and *is* done—by people in their eighties and nineties. Once you learn how to ski, it stays in your bones and muscles forever.

Moving Away from Diabetes

You can begin eliminating the chronic inflammation in your body today. Just pick two movements from this chapter and do them—right now. As you complete each movement, think about how you are fighting the inflammation in every cell within your body. And regardless of which activities you choose to incorporate into your daily life, with every movement you complete, you are working toward a diabetes-free life.

10

Balance

....

Early to bed and early to rise,
makes a man healthy, wealthy, and wise.

—BENJAMIN FRANKLIN (1706–1790)

As humans, we are part of Nature. And in every little cell within our bodies, the force and exuberance of life is at work and following Nature's Laws:

1. Nothing goes to waste.

2. Everything is recycled.

3. Every living being wants to thrive, relish life, and procreate.

4. No one lives forever.

Humans have an inherent consciousness and awareness that life has an end. But to make the most of our short lives, we need The Five Health Essentials. Think of these gifts like a piggy bank of earthly goodies: They are within our reach, waiting to be used. And each of us has the choice to either use them to achieve a more vital life or to waste them.

As a Natural Medicine physician, I believe following The Five Health Essentials has one distinct advantage over all of the popular fad diets and exercise programs currently on the market: There is a focus on obtaining Balance. This Health Essential is the most important one of all, because it reminds you that there are goals in life beyond searching for the perfect diet or having a perfectly sculpted body. To achieve Balance in your life, you should focus on enjoying life to the fullest by filling your days with purpose and meaning. Each day, you should strive to love, learn, share, explore, nurture, care, and create.

Creating a Balanced Life

In Sebastian Kneipp's own words, this Health Essential—Balance—is literally called Order, as in Natural Order. When we accept Nature's laws, we live healthy, full lives. But if we fail to live according to these laws, we tend to think we might be the sole exception—and perhaps these laws don't apply to us. But this isn't true. If you "treat" yourself to a high-fat burger, a milkshake, and some "homemade" apple pie at your favorite restaurant, easily downing all the calories allotted to you for the day in that single meal, you will gain weight; but if you choose healthier fare, you will avoid the weight gain. If you sit on the sofa all day, your muscles will wither; but if you move around during the day (even just a bit), they will become stronger and more toned. And if you show disrespect to important people in your life, you will probably be treated the same way; but if you keep your family together and respect your elders, your children will likely model this behavior.

While everyone has their own definition of balance, this chapter will touch on the essentials of an ordered life. Natural order has nothing to do with the chaos that keeps fun out of your life. The best way to look at Balance is to simply ask yourself: What makes my life good and wonderful?

Balance Basics: Your Six Endowments

For some people, health becomes a new religion. It's all they think about, all they focus on. As you know, I take health very seriously. But other aspects of my life are equally important—and the same should be true for you. Some people say health is the foundation of life, and this is true. But as a physician, I have met many disabled, sickly people who were still full of life and had found usefulness and joy. So while good health is important—and can certainly impact your vitality—there are other equally important areas, such as time, working ability, love and compassion, knowledge, and creativity.

Each of these endowments—including health—can grow and flourish, depending on how you choose to live. If you lose sight of any of these six endowments from Nature, you can lose them. To avoid this, it's important to cherish these gifts and give each the same amount of attention to achieve complete balance, order, and happiness in your life.

Bob's Story

Bob is a teacher who often felt the need to eat in order to make it through his arduous days. He maintained this habit until he realized that not only had he gained weight, but he also felt bloated all the time. And soon, the joints in his fingers and toes hurt constantly. Bob knew his father had developed arthritis in his later years, and he realized how limiting it could be. Finally, when he was diagnosed with type 2 diabetes, he knew something had to change.

Having read about the benefits of an anti-inflammatory, gluten-free diet, Bob decided to give it a shot. Soon after increasing his vegetable intake, he noticed that his arthritis pain had completely disappeared. And since he liked to repair old player pianos to keep some balance in his life, Bob was thrilled to be able to use his fingers again. Though his school work did not leave much time for exercise, he did incorporate little movements through-out his day and focused on using the stairs instead of elevators and parking the car farther away to meet his walking goals each day.

Bob says he never struggled to stick to his new regimen because of the posi-tive feedback he received: Every day he is met with remarks from colleagues and friends about how healthy and happy he looks. But for Bob, the most important benefit is how great he feels. Within just a few months, Bob lost 20 pounds and lowered his A1c from 6.8 to 5.8. He is officially diabetes free and enjoying his life again!

Where to Begin

It's easy to tell someone to find balance, but in this modern world full of hectic schedules and stress, how do you find the time to slow down and live according to Nature's order? Here are a few ways to eliminate stress and find some balance in your life, starting today.

Increase your exposure to sunlight. We are on this planet only by the grace of sunlight: It makes plants grow and synthesizes sugars and starches inside of these plants, and those natural sugars and starches are our essential fuels. After many years of physicians' stern warnings about the dangers of sunlight exposure, we are slowly discovering—or rediscovering—that we need a certain amount of contact with the sun for our well-being. When I was a child, my father—a doctor—would gather neighborhood children and give them a sunbath under hard ultraviolet rays to prevent rickets (a childhood disease that causes the bones to soften). He basically did what tanning booths do now, except not for reasons of beauty.

Today we know that UV rays cause skin cancer, so tanning booths are out. But you should make sure to go out into the sunlight each day so that enough

How Balanced Is Your Life?

When assessing how much balance you currently have—or need—in your life, consider the following questions.

- Do you have a lot of drama and mayhem in your life?
- Are you living within your financial means?
- Do you have a healthy relationship with food?
- Do you start projects and never finish them?
- Are you always having relationship trouble?
- Do you waste water?
- What is your first memory of food?
- Do you have a history of eating disorders?
- Are you patient with children?
- Do you have a tendency to gossip?
- Are you a compulsive overeater? And, conversely, do you eat enough to keep your body nourished?
- Do you think you will be held responsible for your actions at the end of your life?
- What was your first problem with food?
- Are you holding on to old grudges?
- Do you say "please" and "thank you" often?
- What is your family's relationship with food?

vitamin D can be manufactured under your skin. A study found that those with higher levels of vitamin D in their blood were less likely to develop type 2 diabetes.[1] Furthermore, a recent trial showed that by correcting your vitamin D deficiency, you could improve your insulin sensitivity.[2] But it's hard to say exactly how much time you should spend in the sunlight each day. Your local weather forecast usually provides a "UV index" that tells you how much time you can safely spend in the sun. (Make sure to adjust according to your

- Do you use supplements or unnatural products to control your weight?
- How is your relationship with your family?
- Do you watch mindless TV programs?
- Do you reach out to others when you feel lonely?
- Are you always running late?
- Do you ever take time to quietly relax?
- Are you or is anyone else concerned about your eating habits or your weight?
- Do you multitask while you drive?
- Have you given to charity in the last month?
- Are you neighborly?
- Do you work hard to achieve your dreams, or do you think they're out of reach?
- Is your house cluttered?
- Do you recycle?
- Do you lend a helping hand to others—even strangers?
- Do you focus on the problem—or the solution?

If you're not satisfied with your own answers to any of these questions, you should take some time to reflect on ways you can improve those areas in order to create more balance in your life.

skin type: Those with lighter skin should spend less time in direct sunlight.) Start slowly, and make sure to use proper precautions to prevent sunburns: I prefer long-sleeved shirts and a hat to sunscreen lotions that wear off quickly and may come with sides effects.

Keep in mind that your vitamin D requirements can vary. Young skin produces vitamin D more efficiently than older skin. And cloudy days will still help your body create vitamin D, but at a slower rate than when it's sunny outside. Your location—and its distance from the equator—plays a role, as does the smog in your city, which might decrease effective light exposure. Dark skin also decreases the penetration of sunlight (which is the evolutionary purpose of dark skin—to prevent sun damage). So even if you are outside every single day, you could still be low in vitamin D for any of the above reasons. If you suspect that your levels are low in spite of increasing your sun exposure, have your levels checked.

Get more sleep. We do not get enough sleep because we are not in bed very long. And when we are, we toss and turn, getting little or poor-quality sleep. While lack of sleep can lead to crankiness or drowsiness, it can also lead to inflammation—which, as we know, increases your likelihood of developing diabetes, or even cancer. And not getting enough rest causes your stress hormones to rise, which leads to overeating.

If you find that you're having trouble getting enough rest, you might want to try these easy tips.

1. **Go to bed no later than 9:30 p.m.** Remember how we discussed that sleep gives your body a chance to rebuild and repair itself? This repair cycle only lasts from 11:00 p.m. to 1:00 a.m.

2. **Take a book to bed.** Reading something nice before you go to sleep will help to calm and relax you. Avoid thrillers and mysteries, and stick to peaceful writings like poetry.

3. **Make your bedroom as dark as possible.** If you find that you can't avoid light, wear an eye mask. The slightest ray of light—even from your alarm clock—will trigger melatonin-related sensors and will increase restlessness. (So you know what that means: No TV or cell phones, either!)

4. **Keep your feet warm.** If necessary, wear socks to bed or try one of the famous cold-water applications of wet socks: In a sleep study, the one

consistent factor in insomnia was having cold feet, and by wearing cold socks to bed, your body will naturally supply more heat to your feet.

5. **Keep your room cool.** By building a cap with cooling water tubes to keep the brain temperature low, scientists recently discovered that you sleep best when your head is at a little below 60°F. Luckily, you don't need to wear this cap: According to Natural Medicine, you should always sleep with a window open. This will not only keep your head cool, but it will also give you fresh air. Think about it: You don't drink water that has already gone through your body and been discarded. You shouldn't inhale your used-up air, either! And a new study shows that breathing in high levels of carbon dioxide (the gas we exhale after we have inhaled oxygen) decreases mental acuity.[3]

   Ease into this habit by leaving your window open in the spring and summer, when it's warmer outside. By the time the cooler weather begins to set in, you'll be used to having fresh air at night.

6. **Take a natural sleeping aid**—but only as a last resort. If you find that nothing else works, get some hops, valerian, and passionflower capsules. Make sure you alternate the herbs, so as to avoid forming a dependence on any one of them. Most of the time, if you follow the above tips, you will not need them, but it's good to have them on hand. So keep them on your nightstand with a glass of water.

Practice controlled breathing. Health, house, home, hearth, happiness, hope, humor, harmony: These are all positive words that start with an H. The letter H is also the exhaling sound: Hhhh . . . It means we can let go. We don't have to hold our breath because we're worried that something will hit us from behind. We don't have to exert ourselves because we are at home, a place where we can exhale and let out the troubles and worries from the day.

Observe how you are running through your day. Do you find yourself holding your breath in constant fear of a catastrophe hitting? Do you feel stressed and tense most of the time? If so, take control of your breathing—beginning with an exhale: Breathe out for one count, breathe in for one count, breathe out for two counts, breathe in for two counts, and so on until you reach 10 counts. This simple practice takes your mind away from racing thoughts and relaxes your diaphragm, signaling your body that all is well. (It's also another good way to fight insomnia!)

A study performed in 2003 showed that stress increases interleukin-6, a powerful agent of inflammation in the body.[4] But interleukin-6 is not the only chemical in the body that's affected by stress: Stress also creates free radicals that make you age faster. Stress puts your body in high alarm mode via adrenaline and cortisol. And worst of all: It increases abdominal fat, which leads to diabetes and other problems. But did you know that there is bad stress and good stress? Bad stress is what life and other people do to you; good stress comes from setting goals and working hard to achieve them. Life is full of both good stress and bad stress; there's no way to avoid both kinds entirely. So the key here is to find a balance between the two. And the easiest way to start is by taking control of your breathing patterns.

Create your bucket list. In a beautiful children's book titled *Miss Rumphius*, the main character's grandfather lists three things one should achieve in life:

1. Travel to foreign lands.
2. Live at the ocean.
3. Leave the world a more beautiful place.

So are there certain things you want to do or learn, or certain goals you wish to accomplish at some point during your life? If so, write them down now, and begin to tackle that list! Strive for something attainable: You don't want to build your life on fate or luck. Perhaps you'll complete everything on your list, perhaps you won't. The important thing to remember is that by working toward a goal or doing something that interests you, you're on your way to creating balance in your life. And once you've achieved balance, health isn't far behind.

Controlling Stress

There are many methods you can use to control the stress in your life, from decreasing the time you spend alone to simply finding ways to enjoy your downtime. See the list below for a few ideas on reducing the stress in your life.

- **Touch someone.** The more contact you have with the people you love, the better you'll feel. So don't hesitate to reach out to your partner, your child, or your friend. Not only will it give you comfort, but you'll also provide comfort to someone else.

- **Have a pet.** Companionship and contact lower blood pressure and make people live happier, longer lives. So consider getting a pet to keep you company. A cat will show you the wisdom of living a relaxed life, while a dog will always be happy to see you.

- **Get a hobby.** Whether it's music-based, painting, cross-stitching, knitting, or even puttering in the garden, find something that makes you happy—because whatever makes you happy also makes you healthy.

- **Increase your water intake.** A dry cell is a stressed cell. Make sure every cell of your body is hydrated to decrease stress on the cellular level, so that healthy biochemical reactions can take place and sustain your life.

- **Seek joy.** Incorporate as much of this stress reliever into your life as you can. One of the easiest—and most needed—ways to feel joy is by working for the joy of others.

Water

11

Water is the only drink for a wise man.

HENRY DAVID THOREAU (1817–1862)

Water is the most precious molecule of life. We drink it, we bathe in it, and we need it to live. Drinking water reduces inflammation because it facilitates biochemical detoxifying actions within the body. Without it, we would not be able to flush out the waste and toxins in our bodies. But did you know that we can also use water to reduce inflammation in other ways? Whenever cold water hits your skin, it activates a pathway that includes a host of immune modulators, white blood cells, and neurotransmitters that ultimately reduce the inflammation in your body. And when you combine water treatments on the outside of your body with inner hydration, you increase your odds of eliminating the diabetes-causing inflammation from your body.

Water from the Inside

We are mostly water, and, therefore, we need to drink water. We each contain about 5 to 6 liters of blood in our bodies, but that is less than 10 percent of your body weight. In fact, our bodies are made up mostly of water (about 70 percent). And all of this water is in constant flow and turnover, which is why we must stay hydrated by drinking water (or herbal teas): Water supports many biochemical functions. The truth is that we would die quickly without taking a drink—typically within 3 days. Conversely, we can survive without food for about 30 days, on average.

Staying Hydrated

You've probably heard about the importance of staying hydrated, but did you know that you can also drink too much water? I usually recommend that my patients drink about 7 cups of water each day. Seven cups, of course, is an inane recommendation because each body is different—I'm assigning a number merely to keep you mindful of your water intake. Here's how to tell if your water consumption is optimal for your body: Observe your urine. Aim for urine that's slightly yellow in color. If it is getting dark, you need to drink more water. If it is almost clear, you've had too much.

While water is always the best choice for remaining hydrated, soup and fruit also contain nutritious fluids. Coffee and alcoholic drinks such as beer and wine aren't as good for you because they aid in dehydration. But they aren't as unhealthy as hard liquor and milk, which should be avoided altogether due to their inflammatory actions.

To break it down even further, I've included a discussion of the healthiest and unhealthiest beverages you can drink. There's even a short list of beverages that fall in between. But regardless of your preferences, you should never drink anything that's ice cold! Iced liquids hamper digestion by clamping down on blood circulation in your stomach, and they drain energy from your body. Some people reason that the loss of energy helps you lose weight because the cold fluid needs to be warmed in your body, and this process uses up calories. But if you look at it closely, this warming process is not enough to make a serious dent in your weight—though it could be enough to negatively impact your health. Young people, with their abundant energy, might not notice it, but the elderly may feel cold in their middle section and experience lower back pain.

Science also confirms that drinking cold beverages lowers your core temperature.[1] And although studies have shown that cold drinks may improve an athlete's performance in the short term, traditional Chinese medicine (TCM) warns us about the long-term effects. In TCM, cold beverages are discouraged because they diminish your *chi*—your life force.[2]

Healthy Beverages

Water. Stick to filtered, noniced or hot water. An inexpensive pitcher with a renewable filter will remove most heavy metals and germs (if there are any—community tap water is usually very safe in that regard). But you may need to look out for chlorine. Your municipal water works needs chlorine to kill bacteria, but once the water arrives in your home, it's no longer necessary. Chlorine has been linked to asthma, cancer, heart disease, and—wouldn't you know it—diabetes.[3-6] You can get rid of chlorine by letting it evaporate; after 1 day, it is basically all gone. Changing the filter regularly is also of paramount importance, to prevent reintroducing germs.

Herbal (noncaffeinated) teas. Brew your herbal teas yourself because buying them bottled can be expensive (and harmful to the environment). So are there specific herbal teas that are best for you? You can choose based on your preferences because each type offers different plant polyphenols that are beneficial for your health.

Green tea, black tea, and maté tea. All of these teas contain caffeine and antioxidants, and there are many varieties that might suit your palate. Jasmine and rose-scented teas are pleasantly flowery to the palate and don't require sugar.

Garden tea. If you have your own garden, you can use your plants to make seasonal teas by including some dandelions, stinging nettle, and kitchen herbs. You can even throw in some edible leaves—but make sure you do your homework first and learn to discern which parts of a plant are safe to consume.

Hot chocolate. Made without sugar or milk, this requires some getting used to. To transition yourself from standard hot chocolate, try using dark chocolate, almond milk, and stevia. After you reset your taste buds, you will enjoy a nice cup of hot chocolate that provides that touch of pick-me-up you might need in the afternoon. The dark chocolate you'll use is full of antioxidants, too.

Wine. If you have a fatty liver from your diabetes, then you should not drink any alcohol until your liver has recovered. Without taxing a normal liver, the average man can have a glass of wine each day, while a woman can safely have half a glass. Contrary to popular belief, the difference in serving sizes does not have to do with different metabolisms in men and women, but with body size: A taller man has a larger liver than a small woman. So if you are a small man, cut back accordingly. Red wine contains resveratrol, which is touted as the new heal-all and longevity miracle. But resveratrol is only one of thousands of miracle plant compounds that help keep your body healthy—it just happens to be well researched. Grape leaves contain even more resveratrol than red wine does, so consider using them in your garden teas!

Unhealthy Beverages

Milk and dairy-based beverages. Because they promote inflammation—the last thing someone with type 2 diabetes needs—dairy-based beverages should be avoided at all costs.

Soft drinks, including diet drinks. Soft drinks are the number one cause of obesity in this country and contain either sugar (especially fructose) or artificial sweeteners. Fructose, like alcohol, is responsible for fatty liver in diabetics, while artificial sweeteners are suspected to cause side effects, including cancer, obesity, and neurotoxicity. And by consuming artificial sweeteners, you will never lose your sweet tooth and, therefore, will never appreciate the taste of naturally sweet food.

Juices and punches. At the very least, they contain sugars, particularly fructose. Juice adds nothing to your health and actually promotes diabetes because your body does not have to do any work to get the sugar from the juice. (You also miss out on the other nutrients that come from real fruit.) So the next time you think about drinking a glass of apple juice, grab an apple instead!

Sports and energy drinks. Energy comes from making sure your mitochondria—the little energy factories in every cell—are able to work properly. Sports and energy beverages contain sugar, which targets your mitochondria, ultimately triggering the death of your insulin-producing beta cells.[7]

Flavored waters, vitamin waters, and antioxidant-infused beverages. These drinks add nothing to your health. Most of them contain sugars and sweeteners and are not any healthier than soft drinks. You should consume antioxidants and vitamins in their whole forms, from your foods. Why? Artificial antioxidants and vitamins don't work as well as those from a plant because they lack the cofactors needed to process them and protect the cells from a sudden influx of vitamins and antioxidants.

Iced tea. Commercial iced tea drinks are a burden on your stomach and

Tom's Story

"Diabetes runs in my family. My brother has full-blown diabetes and my granddad developed diabetes later in life," says Tom, who knew he was at an increased risk for developing the illness as well. But the Wyoming rancher could never bring himself to give up his diet of beef, bad fats, and soda. "I'd developed poor habits such as eating a large, fat-filled breakfast, big lunches, and big suppers. And I was drinking a lot of soda during the day—definitely more than I ever drank water. I felt completely addicted."

Once Tom was officially diagnosed as prediabetic, he knew something had to change. He decided to stop drinking soda and instead keep himself hydrated with water. It wasn't long before he noticed a change for the better.

"Soon after, my triglyceride levels dropped and my blood sugar began to normalize," he says. "But I still couldn't lose the excess weight." According to Tom, his weight and still-borderline numbers weren't of much concern until he noticed a change in his health. "I began to get persistent joint pain and developed a cough that would last throughout the day."

Eventually, this joint pain led to an extremely painful case of gout. Describing the pain as worse than a broken leg, Tom says he knew it was time to change his diet as well and finally tackle his weight. After consulting with a naturopathic nutritionist, Tom began eating an anti-inflammatory diet.

"In the past 5 months, I've been eating fresh produce, consuming far less meat, gone almost completely off of gluten, and rarely ever consume refined sugar," he says. "Now I don't drink milk or consume any other dairy products."

But that's not all: Tom's family also joined him in his new eating habits—and the results have been astounding. Since the beginning of his journey, Tom has lost a total of 52 pounds, while his wife has lost 35 and his son and daughter-in-law have lost 13 and 25, respectively. Marveling at the changes his family has made, Tom says their diet couldn't be more different today.

"My family doesn't even buy ice cream or cookies anymore," he says. "To tell you the truth, I don't even miss those things because I feel so much better and I've found healthy alternatives that satisfy my cravings."

Another thing Tom doesn't miss: his prediabetes diagnosis. "Since I've started following this plan, I no longer have prediabetes. My weight continues to drop, my cough is gone, I no longer have joint pain, and my energy levels and mobility are drastically improved."

your kidneys, and one of the main ingredients in them is sugar. If you want a summer drink, make a lightly steeped black tea with a handful of dried or fresh mint leaves and drink it without ice.

Bottled water. Bottles burden our Earth. Plus, municipal water works have to adhere to higher standards than bottling operations regarding contaminants, so you might actually be shelling out money for a product that is inferior to your tap water.

Canned or bottled caffeinated beverages. A green or black tea brewed from loose leaves is cheaper and healthier. Most beverages that are purchased contain sugar (which makes them addictive) and are expensive.

Beverages That *Might* Be Healthy (But Require More Research)

Coffee. Traditionally, coffee has been considered unhealthy. If you think about it, coffee is a burned bean, and we talked about how cooking at high heat results in damaging advanced glycation end products (AGEs) in Chapter 5. Coffee is known to raise cholesterol and homocysteine (an inflammation marker). It also raises blood pressure. But surprisingly, new studies have shown that coffee actually benefits your health by reducing your risk of developing type 2 diabetes.[8-9] Even though the effect against diabetes was dose-dependent (the more coffee you drink, the better it is for your diabetes), all of the proof is not yet in, and you should not exceed 3 cups of coffee per day. Certain groups—those with high blood pressure, pregnant women, children, adolescents, and slow caffeine metabolizers—should avoid coffee altogether.

Green coffee. I first encountered green coffee in Saudi Arabia. Instead of burning the beans, the beans in green coffee are ground, made into an infusion, and preserved with cardamom seeds. Served in tiny cups, green coffee tastes much like an herbal tea. It sounds preferable to me—but it has been shown that some of the beneficial polyphenols of the coffee bean are activated only on roasting—and the darker, the better.[10]

Water from the Outside

One of our most important resources on Earth is water. You might not think much of water, but it is actually a very important healing tool. Applying

Revitalizing Your Health with Water

You have numerous opportunities every day to take advantage of the anti-inflammatory powers of water. Below are a few suggestions.

- Splash some cold water on your face first thing in the morning. Not only will this wake you up and increase your energy, but over time it also leaves your skin beautifully toned.

- At the end of your warm shower each day, include a quick cold splash.

- Whenever you visit the restroom, wash your hands with *cold* water (unless you have Raynaud's—a condition where your hands and feet turn white with cold exposure). Contrary to popular belief, warm water irritates your skin and does not kill bacteria better than cold water does.[11] In fact, the effect of cleaning depends only in part on the detergent and more so on the rubbing action and water flow. You might have heard about the *hygiene hypothesis:* We are experiencing more allergies and more infections these days because we are raising our children to be too clean. For those with diabetes, this is no laughing matter, as they are more prone to infection than others.[12]

- Once a week, take a nice warm herbal bath. Warm baths relax and soothe your body, and adding fragrant herbs will only enhance the effects.

- If you live in a warmer climate near an ocean, lake, or river, set aside some time to go for a quick swim.

water to the outside of your body is just as important as having water inside your body. And this is especially true of cold water. When you are exposed to cooler temperatures, it awakens some ancient part of your immune system. Even a modest decrease in room temperature will enhance your well-being. That small bit of cold exposure will use up calories and transform your white fat into brown fat—the kind that helps you lose weight. How does it happen? With the help of a protein called FGF21, which pulls sugars into white cells, where they are turned into energy (instead of just stored, as usual). In effect, FGF21 does the work of insulin—without insulin.[13]

Exposure to cold heals us by causing us to shiver, which produces heat and burns calories. Shivering happens through tiny muscle movements, similar to how exercise produces heat in the body. A short exposure to a cold temperature—like taking a quick cold shower after a hot one—uses this mechanism effectively. But prolonged exposure, like being cold, wet, and miserable all day, might tax the heat production system and lead to a major heat loss, resulting in a drastic drop in core temperature.[14]

Creating a Spa in Your Home

A cold shower or hot herbal bath can turn your unassuming bathroom into a spa. All you need is a tub or shower, a towel, some herbs, and coconut oil.[15] In fact, the word *spa* is an artificial word and derives from the Latin expression *sanitas per aquam*, which means "health through water."

Hot Baths

A hot bath rekindles your metabolic fire, so it is a good idea for diabetics to luxuriate in hot water with healing fragrances. But be careful not to do this too often. Sebastian Kneipp, one of the founders of the Natural Medicine movement and father of hydrotherapy, said that a hot bath a week is a pleasure, but a hot bath every day will weaken your system. Like eating a slice of cake, taking a hot bath is a treat, but bathing in hot water regularly puts you at an increased risk for developing a disease because it reduces your good brown fat. Never immerse yourself in extremely hot bathwater and always end your hot bath with a short cold shower or gush, starting with your feet, followed by your hands, face, and then your whole body. Before you dress or go to bed, slather your skin with coconut oil, which protects your skin from aging, bad germs, and UV light.[16-17] Remove the excess with a paper towel.

Contraindications: A hot bath also lowers your blood pressure, so avoid it if yours is already low; otherwise, it may leave you weak and faint. This may lead to the belief that a hot bath is a remedy for high blood pressure, and this is true—but the effect doesn't last. A cold shower, on the other hand, spikes your blood pressure for a few seconds but lowers it in the long run. If you

Herbs for a Hot Bath

Some herbs just smell good, while others have a medicinal effect. Some herbal baths work through osmosis (some molecules are taken up through your skin) and others by inhaling the healing aromas. Choose your bath herbs according to your needs. And don't be surprised to find that some of the herbs you're using in your foods are also good for bath time!

- Chamomile relieves pain and provides relief from insect bites.
- Dandelion flowers renew your skin and will drive away the winter blues.
- Eucalyptus opens your lungs and helps you breathe.
- Grated ginger enhances bloodflow to all parts of your body.
- Hops relieve insomnia and will leave you sleepy.
- Jasmine enhances your mood and refreshes your skin.
- Lavender calms your nerves and rejuvenates your skin.
- Linden flowers aid in relaxation and could stifle a cold before it takes hold.
- Meadowsweet relieves sore muscles and improves your mood.
- Mint stimulates and heals your skin.
- Orange blossoms aid in relaxation and lower blood pressure.
- Parsley heals bruises.
- Rose petals relax your body and refresh your skin after a long day.
- Rosemary promotes relaxation.
- Sage prevents stiff, sore muscles after a workout.
- Stinging nettle promotes circulation and heals aching joints.

have heart failure or any kind of heart problem, you should avoid hot baths due to the fluid pressure the water exerts on your chest, which can trigger or escalate heart failure. A warm half bath (where the water rises only to your navel) is a good alternative.

USING HERBS

When choosing to take a hot bath, make sure to include healing herbs. There are three different ways you can prepare your herbal baths, depending on your preferences.

1. Throw a handful of herbs directly into the hot bathwater.

2. Brew some herbal tea in a pot, and then add the steeped tea to the bathwater.

3. Buy a commercial herbal bath tea bag, which is much larger than bags used for tea in a cup, and put it into the bathwater. It contains a medley of herbs designed to lift your spirits and soothe your skin. This is an easy way to get the herbs into your bath, but it can be expensive. Also, make sure to avoid any herbs that could cause an allergic reaction. Allergies to herbs are rare, but they can happen.

Cold Showers

After a hot bath, your skin is flushed and warm. As the heat evaporates from your open pores, your body can cool down too much. Taking a short cold shower restores balance by closing your pores. But it does a lot more than that: Cooler bathwater also acts as a stimulant, so try taking a cold shower when you want to go out afterward. See the list below to discover how a cold shower can benefit your health.

WHAT A COLD SHOWER CAN DO FOR YOU

- Boost immune function
- Lift your mood
- Fight fatigue
- Normalize your blood pressure
- Decrease chronic pain
- Improve blood circulation, both arterial and venous
- Detoxify your body
- Deepen breathing, relieving obstructions in your lungs
- Tone subcutaneous connective tissues (that's where modern medicine thinks all the action takes place!)

- Improve lymphatic circulation
- Rejuvenate and heal skin
- Regulate the activity of all glands (pituitary, thyroid, adrenal, ovaries/testes)
- Motivate you to exercise
- Aid in treating diabetes, obesity, gout, rheumatic diseases, chronic fatigue, varicose veins, and hemorrhoids
- Regulate the sympathetic and parasympathetic nervous systems (the nonvoluntary parts of the nervous system) to an optimum

With all of these benefits, you may want to jump into a cold shower right now! But for some people, it is hard to end each warm shower with a cold one. (Of course, it is easier in the summer than in the winter, when water is colder out of the faucet.) Give yourself time for adaptation: Natural Medicine says it can take up to an entire month before you might be ready for a whole-body cold shower (exempting your scalp if it bothers you or if you have sinus problems). Follow the steps below to transition to taking a cold shower at the end of your hot shower or bath.

- After your hot shower, step out of the flow and turn the faucet to cold. Begin by allowing the cold water to hit your feet for a few seconds (I count to six). Then move your hands into the water. Finally, splash your face with the cold water.
- Next time, after you've let the cold water hit your feet, step closer into the running water so that it hits your legs and knees. Follow again with your hands and face. Every time you take a cold shower, let the water hit higher on your body, until you reach your shoulders. (*Note:* If you have sinus problems, do not let the cold water make contact with your scalp, as this can cause sinus pain. Otherwise, it is very invigorating.)
- Here's an extra tip: Exhale! Years ago, I found that exhaling when stepping into cold water helped me to endure it longer. The reason? When you exhale, your body is in a relaxed mode. Conversely, when you inhale, your body goes into alarm mode. Think about it: When we are startled, we suck in our breath. So, by deliberately and slowly exhaling, you're telling your body that everything is all right and there is nothing to fear from the cold water.

Cold Half Bath (Cold Sitz Bath)

A half bath (also known as a sitz bath) can serve as the perfect refreshment on a sweltering summer day and has several health benefits. All you have to do is fill a tub with a few fingers' breadth of cold water and sit there for a minute or two. If you suffer from pelvic ailments, infertility, decreased libido (in both sexes), pelvic pain, chronic prostatitis, leucorrhea, hemorrhoids, or anal fissures, a half bath may offer some relief. A cold bath can also help to reduce varicose veins and relieve insomnia. *Note:* A cold bath is not a good idea if you have an acute urinary tract infection, acute prostatitis, or lower back pain, as your condition may worsen through cold exposure. (Contraindication: Speak with your physician before taking a cold shower if you have uncontrolled high blood pressure, arterial disease, or an acute illness.)

Saltwater Nose Rinse

This water application may sound a bit unappealing at first. But a saltwater nose rinse works well to treat acute colds, acute and chronic sinusitis, hay fever, and sneezing attacks—regardless of their causes. This is because the rinse flushes out your nasal passages, removing dust, pollen, mites, dander, viruses, bacteria, and all kinds of other irritating debris, thereby shortening acute infections and relieving chronic problems like sinusitis, hay fever, and stuffy or dry nose.

To perform the rinse, mix ¼ teaspoon of table or sea salt in a glass of lukewarm water. Stir with a spoon and taste the remaining liquid on the spoon. Its saltiness should be somewhere between that of the ocean and your tears. Now put a bit of the saltwater into your palm and sniff it up one nostril. It may make you feel like you are drowning, but don't panic. Spit out the phlegm that comes down in the back of your throat. Then do the other side. This can be done many times a day, especially when you have an acute cold. For many chronic conditions, do it twice a day. *Note:* I discourage the use of neti pots because they can become contaminated with bacteria. Instead, use your clean, washed hands.

Contraindications: If you tend to have high blood pressure, rinse out your mouth afterward. If the fluid stings or burns your nose, you might have included too little or too much salt, so experiment with your proportions!

Washing Away Diabetes

If water, in its different modalities, can relieve the inflamed bodies of those with type 2 diabetes, why do we hear so little about it? Simply stated, it is much easier to pop a pill than to acknowledge the ancient mechanisms by which our bodies work best. But to reduce the inflammation in your body, it is crucial that you increase your warm water intake and begin administering cold water applications on your skin. And now that you have the tools you need—The Five Health Essentials—you can incorporate these practices into your daily life and finally wave goodbye to your diabetes.

PART 4

Putting It All Together:

Plans, Schedules, and Recipes for Your Healthy Life

12

One Weekend
That Will Change Your Life

··

Don't be afraid to take a big step if one is indicated.
You can't cross a chasm in two small jumps.

—DAVID LLOYD GEORGE (1863–1945)

You've tried them all: the low-carb diet, the high-protein fare, the exercise-only plan. Maybe you've even spent money on workout DVDs you saw on an infomercial. But have any of these methods worked? Have any of those 6- or 8-week promises held true? Or do you struggle to get through each calorie-restricted day, week after week, only to indulge in pastries and other comfort foods when you have an especially tough day?

If this sounds familiar, it's time to say goodbye to your old ways of thinking. You've realized those fad diets and extreme workouts don't work and that it takes a true lifestyle change to reduce diabetic inflammation. And now that you're armed with the knowledge of how The Five Health Essentials can heal your inflamed body, there's nothing holding you back from curing your diabetes for good!

The Weekend Jump Start

Surprise: You can begin to cure your diabetes—and reclaim your health—in a single weekend. I know what you're thinking: "Why should I give up my weekend? That's *my* time. I'll start on Monday." And you're right—it *is* your time. So why not use it to do something good for yourself? Plus, polls have shown that starting a new health plan during the weekend actually increases your odds of sticking with it, because you're not overwhelmed by your work responsibilities and you have time to focus on yourself. By getting in the right mind-set over the weekend, you mentally prepare yourself to make time for your health during the workweek.

Friday Evening

If you work all week, it is a good idea to start your new, healthy life on a Friday night, when you won't have the stress of rising early for work the next day. So here are your tasks to complete when you get home on Friday.

1. **Brew yourself an herbal tea.** Use whatever herbs or spices you have in the house—like peppermint or chamomile—to make an herbal tea. Keep it easy and quick. Sip your tea as you do your evening chores, and try to finish it before dinner. If you don't have the ingredients to make an herbal tea, drink water.

2. **Play some music.** Choose something that's soothing or uplifting. Stay away from loud, aggressive music: The point is to relax after your long day and to bring balance into your life. And try to stay away from the TV, computer, and phone—for now.

3. **Do some knee bends.** Try to complete 21 knee bends, but only do what you can. If you experience any trouble, you can substitute one of the movements listed in Chapter 9.

4. **Make a simple meal for dinner.** Tonight you won't have time to cook, but you should be eating something healthy to fight your diabetes. So whether you have some leftovers from earlier in the week or you choose to bring home some takeout, keep your dinner preparation quick. Just make sure it's as healthy as possible, like avocado sushi, or some sautéed vegetables and a piece of fish or meat, or a salad fortified with protein. And make sure you're not trying to "diet": Eat enough to make sure you're satisfied, and have some fruit for dessert.

5. **Set the table as if you're expecting company.** If you have a family, let your children or your spouse help. By using your nicest dishes and even including a simple centerpiece (if you have one) or some candles and flowers, you're placing importance on yourself. Why should you save your best dishes and decorations for company? This is a special occasion: Today, you're beginning your new life! Lay down the new rules. If your family does not plan to join you in this new lifestyle, that's okay—you can be confident that one day they will follow your lead.

6. **Serve dinner.** Before you begin eating, take three deep breaths or take a moment to appreciate all that you have. (And make sure to turn off the music so that you can eat your dinner without distractions.)

7. **Put down your fork or spoon after each bite.** Chew slowly, and pay attention to what you are eating. If you have company, you can discuss common interests in between bites. (You may want to talk about the changes you are going to implement, starting tonight.) Don't allow TV, games, or other distractions at the table. Take your time and enjoy your meal.

8. **Do the dishes.** If you have a family, ask someone else to do the dishes because nobody should have to cook *and* do the dishes. If you live alone and you're tired from your commute home, soak your dishes in the sink and wash them the next morning.

9. **Go for a short walk around the block.** If you have a family, feel free to take them along. But you can also use this time for self-reflection or to congratulate yourself for making this positive change in your life. If you can't walk tonight, choose another movement to complete from Chapter 9.

10. **Grab a big trash bag and clean out your refrigerator.** Take your time and read the labels on your foods. Use Chapter 7 as a guide for what to keep and what to toss. And when in doubt, toss it out! (Prepackaged and labeled items are suspect.) When you're finished, wipe down the shelves.

11. **Take some time for yourself.** Whether you want to watch TV, spend quality time with your partner or family, or jump on the computer, take some time to relax. But make sure you stay aware of the time so you don't stay up too late.

12. **Groom for the night.** Do a quick, cold, whole-body wash with a washcloth in front of the sink or standing in the tub. If you prefer to take a warm shower or a hot herbal bath (provided you have herbs in

your house), end it with a cold burst of water. And as you brush your teeth, stand on one leg, and then the other.

13. **Go to bed with a book.** If you have a book or magazine you've wanted to read, now is the perfect time. Just make sure it's something calming. Reading a mystery or thriller may make it hard to fall asleep. Playing soft music will help you relax, but leave all other electronics turned off. In fact, consider moving your TV out of your bedroom; having a TV in the bedroom has been linked to a sedentary lifestyle and obesity.[1]

So let's assess what you did in a single evening on the new program.

Water. You ended either your hot bath or warm shower with a burst of cold water or washed your entire body with cold water, which strengthened your immune system and helped to maintain your motivation.

Movement. You did two mini-exercises (or one mini-exercise and a walk). You also stood on one leg while brushing your teeth, which strengthened your muscles and bones, reduced your blood sugar, and lowered your insulin resistance. In addition, you moved around in your kitchen while ridding your refrigerator of toxic food.

Food. You ate a healthy meal, thereby nudging your metabolism in a new direction—toward healing.

Herbs. You drank an herbal tea and possibly had an herbal bath, healing your cells in the process.

Balance. You decluttered part of your house (your refrigerator). During dinner, you slowed down and practiced mindfulness and gratitude. And you went to bed early to prepare for a good and productive day tomorrow. Remember: Getting plenty of sleep reduces the stress hormone cortisol, gives your immune system a chance to repair damaged DNA, and reduces inflammation.

Saturday

1. **Take a warm shower, ending with a quick cold one.**

2. **Eat an anti-inflammatory breakfast.** Given that you have to use what you have in your house, it can be two boiled eggs and an apple or an orange. Or you can eat two eggs sunny-side up with one strip of bacon. (You shouldn't eat bacon regularly, but you may have it on occasion. For example, when I travel and have to eat in hotels, I choose eggs and

bacon because they are far healthier for my metabolism than sweetened cereals, inferior breads, and dubious dairy products.)

3. **Clean out your freezer and pantry,** and write a shopping list for replacement items. Again, make sure to read the labels on your foods to check for hidden inflammatory toxins. Only keep food that furthers your cause. (Sure, that can of icing may be brand-new, but if it only inflames your cells and promotes your diabetic state, is it really worth it?) When you're finished, wipe down the shelves and organize the remaining products.

4. **Take a trip to your local supermarket.** See "Your Shopping List" on page 186 for a list of foods to get you started.

5. **Stow your purchases** in your pantry, fridge, and freezer.

6. **Eat lunch.** Using the foods you just purchased, make yourself an anti-inflammatory lunch. Perhaps a quick salad from greens, fresh or dried anti-diabetic herbs, black pepper, salt, a few nuts or a can of sardines (or shrimp), and either olive oil or a spoonful of mayonnaise. Or skip ahead to Chapter 14 for some easy, delicious recipes.

7. **Relax.** Now that you've stocked your kitchen for the next week and eaten your lunch, take time to enjoy your weekend. Go ahead and spend a few hours catching up with friends and family, or go watch that movie that was just released in the local theater. This is your time to do whatever it is that you enjoy.

8. **Take a walk.** It's important to get outside while there's still daylight so you get your daily dose of vitamin D. Even if it is raining, walk around your neighborhood or even just around your block. Try to spend at least 10 minutes outdoors today.

9. **Prepare dinner.** Tonight you'll prepare a wonderful, filling (and easy!) dinner. Remember to include two or three vegetables, a small amount of protein, and some good fats. Here's a suggestion: Pan-fried fish with herbs in coconut oil, leafy greens sautéed with olive oil and garlic, and a garden salad with tomatoes, fresh herbs, and olive oil. Treat yourself to some fresh fruit for dessert.

10. **Repeat steps 5 through 8 from Friday night.** It's important to get into the habit of setting your table for every single meal as a reminder of your new lifestyle.

11. **Do a 1-minute movement from Chapter 9.** You can choose any movement or activity that appeals to you, but try to incorporate some exercise into your evening. You can even do your movement while watching TV or sitting on the sofa with your partner.

12. **Repeat steps 11 through 13 from Friday night.** Ending your evening with relaxation and quality time with your family will provide the balance you've been seeking.

Your Shopping List

The food listed below is enough to feed one person for an entire week. (And some items, such as the olive oil, will last quite a bit longer.) If you have a family, you'll need to shop for more vegetables, fish, and meat.

- A bottle of **olive oil,** preferably virgin and organic
- A jar of **virgin coconut oil**, preferably organic
- One or two bulbs of **garlic** and/or dried garlic powder
- A bag of **onions**
- **Two green leafy vegetables** (kale, dinosaur kale, red or green chard, cabbage leaves, etc.)
- **One head of cauliflower**, preferably organic
- **Two root vegetables**, such as red beets and carrots
- **One head of lettuce**—anything from romaine to Belgian chicories or whatever you like
- **Herbs** like parsley, dill, and cilantro—fresh if you can get them, dried (whole or ground) if you cannot
- **Brown rice** and/or **green lentils** (also called French or Champagne lentils)
- **Fresh fruit,** like an apple, pear, or orange for dessert each day. Stay away from dried, canned, or processed fruit.
- **Ocean fish,** like herring, cod, hake, smelt, or mackerel. Whatever you buy, it should not be farm-raised or freshwater fish as they contain less of the healthy omega-3 oils.

Sunday

You should follow the same steps on Sunday that you did on Saturday, with a few additions:

1. **Use your morning for a spiritual practice.** Take a walk in Nature, do some yoga, or attend a religious service.

2. **Go outdoors.** If you haven't done so already, go for a walk, bike ride, or hike, preferably with family or friends. In the future, you might want to find like-minded groups such as bird watchers, herbalists, or hikers.

- **Raw sunflower seeds** (or other raw seeds or nuts like flaxseeds, walnuts, almonds, pecans, and hazelnuts)

- One can of **organic beans** for breakfast. (Eden is the only brand without BPA.)

- Alternatively, you can grab **breakfast cereal** from the bulk bin— like gluten-free granola, European-style muesli, or a package of rolled oats—but no packaged commercial cereals.

- If you opt for cereal, you may need *organic unsweetened* **soy, hemp, almond,** or **rice milk.**

- One carton of **organic eggs**

- One can of **sardines** in water, preferably *with* bones

- **Salt**—kosher is the cheapest and is usually not adulterated. Sea salt is fine, unless nonclumping agents have been added. They may contain sugars or aluminum!

- **Black pepper**

- **Chicken, turkey, lamb, or ground beef,** if you want to cook meals for several days. The meat needs to be *organic* and/or *USDA-approved, grass-fed.*

- Optional: A jar of organic olive oil mayonnaise

3. **Cook for the week.** To save yourself some time during your busy workweek, plan your meals ahead of time and cook some food for the week. Bear in mind that not everything needs to be prepared ahead of time because sautéing some vegetables in olive oil or pan-frying a fish fillet will only take a few moments. But if you're making a meat loaf or some small homemade hamburgers with herbs, garlic, and olive oil, that may take longer—and these dishes can be frozen easily. Separate the food into daily portions and freeze them. When you're done, you can sit back and relax, knowing you've reduced your workload for the next 5 days. And if you're struggling to develop a meal plan for the next week, turn to the next chapter. I've provided 2 weeks' worth of menus, along with a daily outline of how to incorporate each of The Five Health Essentials to get you started.

13

The First Steps in Your
Diabetes-
Free Life

···

Our greatest happiness does not depend on
the condition of life in which chance
has placed us but is always the result
of a good conscience, good health,
occupation, and freedom in all just pursuits.

—THOMAS JEFFERSON (1743–1826)

You've made it through the weekend, which means you've begun to change
your life and reduce that harmful, toxic inflammation inside of your body.
Congratulations! Maybe you're already feeling the positive effects of your
new lifestyle. But now it's Sunday night, and perhaps you're questioning how
you're going to be able to maintain this new lifestyle. Weekdays bring along
more stress, less free time, and a whole new set of responsibilities. And if
you're a voracious carnivore or have a big sweet tooth, you're probably wondering how you're going to be able to cut down on those items to make room
for all those filling, anti-inflammatory vegetables.

Taking all of this into account, I've provided a 2-week sample plan to get you started. Think of the weekend as your jump start: You focused on getting your kitchen, your mind, and maybe even your family ready for this lifestyle change. Now it's time to make it a habit.

When you look at the plan below, you'll notice that Week 1 is designed to help you transition into your new lifestyle while juggling the demands of your workday or weekly obligations. Week 2 serves to push you a little further by helping you gradually increase your movements and herbal intake each day while you're slowly reducing your meat intake. And both weeks contain dishes (shown in italics) that are accompanied by recipes in Chapter 14.

Use this plan as a guideline—and remember that each body and circumstance is different, so customize it as needed. Perhaps you have extra time to cook fresh meals for each day of the week and you already walk every day. Or maybe your time is limited and you need to incorporate leftovers more often in order to fit in your daily movements. Whatever the case, your goal is to ultimately include six movements throughout the day while having 3 meat- and fish-free days each week. It may take you longer than 2 weeks to accomplish this—and that's okay! The important thing is that you remain committed.

Try to complete each of The Five Health Essentials to the best of your ability. If you miss one, don't worry; just be sure to do it the next day. Every completed task is a step toward your diabetes-free life. And reminding yourself of this every day will give you the hope, motivation, and confidence you need in order to stick with it for the long run. So welcome to your new life: You're officially on the road to receiving *your* diabetes-free diagnosis!

WEEK 1: Transitioning from Weekend to Weekday

MONDAY

FOOD

Breakfast: Rolled oats with ½ cup fresh berries and your choice of soy, hemp, almond, or rice milk; herbal tea

Lunch: Grilled hamburger and a green salad with tomatoes, fresh herbs, and olive oil. (You may also purchase your lunch during the first few days on this plan until you're used to cooking in advance. Just remember: Whatever you buy for lunch should be anti-inflammatory and healthy!)

Dinner: Baked fish fillet with *Lemony Beet Greens* (page 213), parsnips, and brown rice

Dessert: A fresh apple or, if you want something more, try *Baked Apples* (page 262)

HERBS

Drink another cup of herbal tea before dinner. Incorporate at least one anti-diabetic herb or spice into your meals.

MOVEMENT

Choose two 1-minute movements to complete today. If you're extremely busy, try to sneak them into your day, like when you're stuck at your desk or when you're engaged in a phone conversation. Also, take a 10-minute walk outside. You can either walk during your lunch break or in the evening, after dinner. And don't be afraid to ask for company: Walking with a friend, colleague, or spouse will help the time go by faster. (Bonus: This will also count toward your Balance goals for the day!)

BALANCE

Because this is your first day back at work, it's important to make sure you stay on track. Clean your work space in honor of your new start. Set your table for dinner each night, just as you did on Saturday and Sunday. And before you go to bed, spend some quality time with your family or touch base with an old friend.

WATER

Take a cold shower or end your warm shower with a cold burst. And if you shower in the morning, wash your body at night with some cold water. Try to stay aware of your fluid intake throughout the day, and drink at least 7 cups of warm or room-temperature water. (Remember: No ice!)

TUESDAY

FOOD
Breakfast: Granola with a sliced apple or pear and your choice of soy, hemp, almond, or rice milk; green tea
Lunch: Romaine salad with avocado, fresh (or dried) garden herbs, olive oil, salt, and pepper; add a small piece of meat or fish for extra protein
Dinner: *Herbal Soup* (page 228) with ground beef and vegetables
Dessert: Mangoes topped with *Whipped Coconut Cream* (page 269)

HERBS
Drink a cup of herbal tea before dinner. Incorporate one or two anti-diabetic herbs or spices into your meals.

MOVEMENT
Choose two 1-minute movements to complete today. If you struggled with a particular movement yesterday, try to do it again. Make sure not to forget your daily 10-minute walk.

BALANCE
Do you like to sing, write, read, paint, or draw? Or perhaps there's another activity or hobby you enjoy. Don't start yet—but think about what you might enjoy doing and create a plan to make this activity part of your life. Also, think of a way you can help bring joy to others. Does your elderly neighbor need a hand with shopping? Is the lady next to you at the supermarket struggling with her bags? Reach out and offer to help.

WATER
Take a cold shower or end your warm shower with a cold burst. Make sure to stay hydrated during the day.

WEDNESDAY

FOOD
Breakfast: *Breakfast Beans* (page 225), an apple, and herbal tea
Lunch: *Potato, Kale, and Leek Soup* (page 213) and a small take-out salad
Dinner: Vegetarian dinner of mushrooms, carrots, parsnips, peas, and brown rice
Dessert: 1 cup fresh berries sprinkled with chocolate nibs or chips

HERBS
Drink another cup of herbal tea before dinner, using a different herb from the night before. Incorporate one or two anti-diabetic herbs or spices into your meals.

MOVEMENT
Choose three 1-minute movements to complete today. You can repeat the same moves from yesterday or mix it up a bit. In fact, you can even multitask by doing the Walking Side Step movement (page 148) during your walk!

BALANCE
Wake up 5 minutes earlier to meditate, exercise, or simply walk barefoot in the grass. It's now the middle of the week, and odds are you're feeling a little tired. So tonight, try to go to bed an hour earlier than usual. You've had a busy few days, so curl up in bed with a good book. You may even want to begin journaling about your new journey. Don't be afraid to say "lights out" before the rest of your family.

WATER
Is that cold burst at the end of your warm shower getting easier? And how's your fluid intake? In addition to observing the color of your urine, you can make sure your water exposure and hydration needs are being met by keeping track of your progress in a journal or notebook.

THURSDAY

FOOD

Breakfast: Two eggs sunny-side up, fresh sliced avocado, an orange, and green tea

Lunch: Grilled hamburger, fresh carrots with ghee and dill, and a green salad with tomatoes, fresh herbs, and olive oil

Dinner: *Shrimp Salad* (page 254) with fresh mandarin oranges, red beets, and mixed greens with olive oil and vinegar

Dessert: *Crustless Apple Pie* (page 263)

HERBS

Drink a cup of herbal tea before dinner. Incorporate one or two anti-diabetic herbs or spices into your meals.

MOVEMENT

Choose three 1-minute movements to complete today. Are certain moves becoming easier? Hopefully, your daily walk is now a natural part of your routine. But if you're struggling to fit it in, try breaking it up into 5-minute increments. Sometimes it's easier to find 5 spare minutes twice a day than it is to block out a larger amount of time. Make your new lifestyle work for you!

BALANCE

Is there something you've been wanting to do for a while, but you "don't have the time"? When you get home this evening, create a plan to make it happen! While it's important to meet the demands of your daily schedule, you also need to create time for your dreams. So go to that new exhibit or sign up for that sewing class down at the neighborhood center. You may even want to learn a new language or play a musical instrument. Do whatever it is you desire. And give yourself a big pat on the back for making yourself a priority!

WATER

Take a cold shower or end your warm shower with a cold burst. Be mindful today whenever you wash your hands—are you using cold water instead of warm? And at dinner, try to recall how many cups of water or herbal tea you drank today.

FRIDAY

FOOD
Breakfast: Rolled oats with apples, cinnamon, and your choice of soy, hemp, almond, or rice milk; herbal tea
Lunch: *Potato, Kale, and Leek Soup* (page 213) and a small take-out salad
Dinner: Baked fish fillet with *Lemony Beet Greens* (page 213), shredded red beets, and quinoa
Dessert: Fresh pineapple slices with *Whipped Coconut Cream* (page 269)

HERBS
Drink another cup of herbal tea before dinner. Incorporate one or two anti-diabetic herbs or spices in your meals.

MOVEMENT
Choose three 1-minute movements to complete today. Make one of them the Arm Extensions (page 149), and do it during your walk.

BALANCE
Today, make a list of everything positive you have in your life. By reflecting on all of your blessings, you'll develop a new appreciation for those you hold dear. And think about why you were put in this life—and what you can learn from it.

WATER
Start your day with a cold shower, or end your warm shower with a cold burst. At the end of the day, take a hot herbal bath to help you unwind from your busy week.

SATURDAY

FOOD
Breakfast: *Breakfast Beans* (page 225), sliced cantaloupe, and green tea
Lunch: Romaine salad with quinoa, avocado, fresh or dried garden herbs, olive oil, salt, and pepper
Dinner: *Herbal Soup* (page 228) with ground beef and vegetables
Dessert: *Chocolate-Covered Banana* (page 262) or a banana sautéed in ghee and sprinkled with cinnamon

HERBS
Drink a cup of herbal tea today while reading or watching TV. Try to incorporate an anti-diabetic herb into each of your meals.

MOVEMENT
It's now the weekend, and you have a little more time on your hands, so choose either four 1-minute movements or an outdoor activity to complete today, in addition to your daily walk. And if you complete your 10-minute walk and want to go for a longer stroll, keep going!

BALANCE
So what did you plan to do this weekend? Perhaps you have an outing with friends or a date with your partner. Use this time to reconnect with the important people in your life. (But make sure to set aside some time for yourself, too! Consider setting aside 5 minutes to meditate and clear your mind.)

WATER
Take a cold shower or end your warm shower with a cold burst. Weekends can get busy, but it's still important to keep track of your water intake. Now's not the time to become dehydrated.

SUNDAY

FOOD
Breakfast: *Fruit Smoothie* (page 264)
Lunch: *Easy Arugula Salad with Egg* (page 216)
Dinner: Vegetarian dinner of mushrooms, carrots, parsnips, peas, and quinoa
Dessert: *Marinated Peaches* (page 264)

HERBS
Drink a cup of herbal tea midmorning. Try to incorporate an anti-diabetic herb into each of your meals today.

MOVEMENT
Choose four 1-minute movements to complete today. If you chose to take a longer walk yesterday and feel a little sore, you can cut your daily walk back by a few minutes today. Make sure you listen to your body and don't push yourself too hard.

BALANCE
Linger in bed for a few moments and make a plan for the day. Toss out all negative thoughts and situations. Strive for a happy day. Have a spiritual practice in place, even if it just means lighting a candle and meditating or saying a prayer of thanks. Plan your meals for the following week and shop for what you need. When you return from the supermarket, take a few moments to relax before you begin cooking. You may even want to sit outside for a few moments to enjoy the sounds of Nature.

WATER
Take a cold shower or end your warm shower with a cold burst. And drink some water while you're in the kitchen cooking next week's meals.

WEEK 2: Embracing The Five Health Essentials

MONDAY

FOOD

Breakfast: Granola with organic blueberries and your choice of soy, hemp, almond, or rice milk; green tea
Lunch: Baked fish fillet with sautéed kale and baked sweet potato
Dinner: Herbed turkey with your choice of two vegetables
Dessert: 1 cup fresh cherries

HERBS

Drink a cup of herbal tea before dinner. Incorporate one or two anti-diabetic herbs or spices into each of your meals.

MOVEMENT

Choose four 1-minute movements to complete today and plan them around your schedule. If you work at a desk, try to sneak in a few during the day, when you need a break.

BALANCE

Remember the hobby or activity you chose last Tuesday? Set aside time today to make sure you're following through with your action plan. If you can find the time during the week, try to spend at least a few minutes each day working on something you enjoy. And at the very least, set aside an hour or two each week to keep up with your new activity.

WATER

Take a cold shower or end your warm shower with a cold burst. If you suffer from varicose veins or insomnia, try taking a short, cold sitz bath at night before you go to bed.

TUESDAY

FOOD
Breakfast: Baked sweet potato topped with hummus; an orange; green tea
Lunch: *Chard and Chickpea Stew* (page 211)
Dinner: Vegetarian dinner of *Curried Spaghetti Squash* (page 226), *Roasted Baby Potatoes* (page 233), steamed collards, and mushrooms
Dessert: 1 cup fresh berries with *Whipped Coconut Cream* (page 269)

HERBS
Drink a cup of herbal tea before dinner. Incorporate one or two anti-diabetic herbs or spices into each of your meals.

MOVEMENT
Choose five 1-minute movements to incorporate into your day. If you have a hard time remembering to fit them all in, you can set an alarm on your phone as a reminder until it becomes second nature.

BALANCE
Today, take a few moments to write in your journal. If you don't have one, a notebook or some scrap paper will do. Focus on writing down your dreams. Do you have any goals that you want to achieve? Are there any milestones you want to reach within the next year? Choose goals you can work toward versus those that may be unattainable. Keep this record in a safe place and read it at least once a week to stay on track.

WATER
Take a cold shower or end your warm shower with a cold burst. By now, your tolerance for cold water should be a little higher. Have you noticed that it's getting easier? And how's your water intake? If you've been hydrating yourself properly, you may be noticing a change in your skin as well as your energy level.

WEDNESDAY

FOOD

Breakfast: Two hard-cooked eggs with sautéed greens, peaches, and herbal tea
Lunch: Garden salad with avocado, cucumber, an assortment of chopped vegetables, oil, and vinegar
Dinner: *Herbed Lamb Chops* (page 244) with spinach, asparagus, summer squash, and mashed cauliflower
Dessert: *Pineapple Mousse* (page 264)

HERBS

Drink another cup of herbal tea before dinner. Incorporate one or two anti-diabetic herbs or spices into each of your meals.

MOVEMENT

Do five 1-minute movements or, if you've built up enough strength, try to do one of the Five Tibetan Rites today. Keep in mind that the Rites are more difficult to complete than the 1-minute movements, so if you're experiencing trouble, adapt the Rites to make them easier. Remember: Avoiding injury is more important than perfecting each movement.

BALANCE

It's Wednesday again, which means it's time to get into bed an hour earlier than you usually do. If you have trouble falling asleep, play some music or read a good book, which will help you relax. And make sure to forgive and forget any grievances. As Ralph Waldo Emerson said, "Finish every day and be done with it."

WATER

Take a cold shower or end your warm shower with a cold burst. Remember to avoid your scalp if you have sinus troubles.

THURSDAY

FOOD
Breakfast: Granola with ½ cup organic strawberries and coconut milk; herbal tea
Lunch: Egg salad wrap in lettuce leaves
Dinner: Vegetarian dinner of *Vegetable Stir-Fry* (page 234), mixed greens, and *Roasted Baby Potatoes* (page 233)
Dessert: *Chocolate-Covered Banana* (page 262)

HERBS
Drink another cup of herbal tea before dinner. Incorporate one or two anti-diabetic herbs or spices into each of your meals.

MOVEMENT
Do five 1-minute movements or try a couple of the Tibetan Rites today. You can always mix a few of your 1-minute movements with one or two of the Rites if you need to take it slow.

BALANCE
Set aside 10 minutes tonight to declutter your home. We all have one surface or corner in our house that needs special attention. Maybe it's where your mail collects, or maybe you simply need to reorganize a cabinet. Either way, you'll feel better knowing that your home is a little more organized. When you're done, spend some time with your family or a good book.

WATER
Take a cold shower or end your warm shower with a cold burst. Are you still drinking enough water? Keeping yourself hydrated is essential if you want to reduce the inflammation in your body.

FRIDAY

FOOD
Breakfast: *Breakfast Beans* (page 225), and apple, and green tea
Lunch: Fresh take-out salad or soup
Dinner: Herb-roasted turkey with your choice of two vegetables
Dessert: *Marinated Peaches* (page 264)

HERBS
Drink a cup of herbal tea before dinner. Incorporate one or two anti-diabetic herbs or spices into each of your meals.

MOVEMENT
Try to complete six 1-minute movements today and walk for at least 10 minutes. While you're walking, take a few moments to reflect on everything you've done in the last 2 weeks to begin reversing your diabetes.

BALANCE
Whether it's by phone, social media, or in person, take some time to reconnect with old friends. Don't let your busy life get in the way of your important relationships. You may also want to put aside some time to think about where you're headed or what you've done in the past. Write your life story as if it were a funny movie. Then rewrite it as if it were a Shakespearean drama. Looking at your life from two different perspectives may help with reflection.

WATER
Is your cold water routine slowly becoming second nature? Keep it up! At the end of the night, take a hot herbal bath to help you unwind from the week.

SATURDAY

FOOD
Breakfast: *Vegetable Smoothie* (page 265)
Lunch: *Chard and Chickpea Stew* (page 211)
Dinner: Baked fish fillet with sautéed kale and baked sweet potato
Dessert: 1 cup organic strawberries topped with melted dark chocolate

HERBS
Drink a cup of herbal tea midmorning. Try to incorporate one or two anti-diabetic herbs into each of your meals.

MOVEMENT
Choose six 1-minute movements to complete today. Aim to complete three movements before lunch. If you're ready for a bigger challenge, you can begin the Zen running program on page 153 in place of your daily walk.

BALANCE
What's the one area of your life that requires the most improvement (outside of having diabetes)? Maybe you are always running late or tend to lose patience quickly. Whatever your struggle, brainstorm ways you can improve this area of your life—and start working on it today!

WATER
Take a cold shower or end your warm shower with a cold burst. And make sure you're staying hydrated throughout the weekend.

SUNDAY

FOOD

Breakfast: Omelet with sautéed onions, asparagus, and fresh herbs; herbal tea
Lunch: *Easy Arugula Salad with Egg* (page 216)
Dinner: Vegetarian dinner of *Curried Spaghetti Squash* (page 226), *Roasted Baby Potatoes* (page 233), asparagus, steamed collards, and mushrooms
Dessert: *Crustless Apple Pie* (page 263)

HERBS

Drink a cup of herbal tea midmorning. Use anti-diabetic herbs freely in each meal.

MOVEMENT

Either complete six 1-minute movements or go outside and work in your garden for half an hour. If you've been walking alone for the past 2 weeks or just started Zen running, try to recruit your partner or a neighbor to come along with you. Not only will you be getting some exercise, but you'll also be halfway to meeting your balance goals for the day.

BALANCE

It's time to plan, shop for, and prepare next week's meals. While you're cooking, play some soothing music in the background. If you're craving some quality time with your spouse, ask him or her to help you out in the kitchen. Planning the meals together will not only make your partner feel included in your new lifestyle, but it will also help you to stay connected. And try to get to bed a little earlier tonight: You've done a lot to benefit your health in the past 2 weeks, so get the rest you need.

WATER

By now, you should be craving your cold water morning routine. If you can fit it into your day (and have access to a body of water), try to go for a short swim today. Not only will you benefit from the anti-inflammatory powers of the water, but you'll also be able to enjoy a few extra moments of relaxation while helping your body decrease its insulin resistance.

A Cooking Course for
Easy Dishes

No disease that can be treated by diet
should be treated with any other means.

—MOSES MAIMONIDES (1135-1204)

In a country where most kitchens look like designs from movie sets and people read cookbooks like they're mysteries, few actually cook a warm meal every day. Whether it's because they never learned basic cooking skills or simply feel they just don't have enough time to make a homemade meal, many are depending on inflammatory take-out food or, even worse, fast food to satisfy their hunger pangs. But without home-cooking, the diabetes epidemic in the United States will never end, so here's some good news: If you think you don't have the time to cook, or you don't know where to begin in the kitchen, I'm here to guide you.

This chapter is full of easy cooking charts that include instructions and quick cooking tips for everything from steaming vegetables and braising meat to whipping up quick salads and choosing fresh fruit. And if you have more time on the weekends and want to challenge yourself, I've also included some delicious recipes to provide more variety. So get ready to dive in: Here is your mini-cooking course, as easy as 1-2-3.

Items You'll Need

There are some essential pieces of cooking equipment and utensils—along with a small variety of herbs and spices—you'll need in order to get started.

- A midsize stainless steel skillet with a lid
- A stainless steel, ovenproof skillet. If you have only one, midsize is best. (Extra points if it's deep, since it can serve several purposes.)
- A stainless steel spatula
- Kitchen knives: A small paring knife and a large, sturdy kitchen, or chef's, knife
- A vegetable peeler (you could also use a small kitchen knife for the same purpose)
- Virgin, unrefined coconut oil, preferably organic
- Olive oil, preferably organic
- Black pepper, ground
- Salt (sea salt or Kosher salt are best)
- Garlic, dry or fresh (Don't opt for jarred garlic that's already minced or peeled—it spoils fast.)
- Dried herbs: There are so many, and you will slowly add more as you need them. But start with dill, parsley, oregano, basil, Italian seasoning, and herbes de Provence.

Greens

Because they contain the most anti-diabetic phytonutrients of all vegetables, greens are the best foods you can put on your plate. The chart below features a selection of healthy greens, along with simple instructions for prep and cooking suggestions.

Greens	Weight (4–6 Cooked Servings)	Prep	Cooking Methods	Approximate Cooking Times	Cooking Suggestions
Beet greens	1½–2 pounds	Wash thoroughly, cut in strips.	Young greens can be eaten raw, steamed, or sautéed.	5–10 minutes	Season with sea salt, black pepper, ghee or olive oil, vinegar, chives, and dill.
Chard (called Italian spinach)	1½–2 pounds	Wash and cut in strips.	Steam or sauté in olive oil, garlic, salt, and pepper.	10 minutes	Cook with white beans and garlic; use in soups; sauté with onion and garlic in olive oil or ghee, and season with hot peppers, crushed red pepper, or just black pepper and mustard seeds; serve with brown rice.
Collards	1½–2 pounds	Wash and cut in strips.	Steam, boil, or sauté in olive oil, garlic, salt, and pepper.	5–15 minutes	Cook with pork or other vegetables in coconut oil, olive oil, or ghee with garlic and onion or chopped tomatoes; season with sea salt, black pepper, and paprika.

Greens	Weight (4–6 Cooked Servings)	Prep	Cooking Methods	Approximate Cooking Times	Cooking Suggestions
Dandelion	1½–2 pounds	Wash leaves thoroughly.	Use in salads, steam, or boil. Delicious with olive oil, garlic, salt, and black pepper.	5–10 minutes	Best cooked with onions and garlic in a stock. Good combined with stinging nettles.
Grapevine leaves	A handful of leaves	Wash and remove stems.	Steaming is best. Delicious with olive oil, garlic, salt and black pepper.	3–5 minutes	Add a few leaves to other greens.
Kale, Tuscan or dinosaur	1½–2 pounds	Rinse thoroughly.	Slightly bitter when eaten raw; steam, or boil. Delicious with olive oil, garlic, salt, and black pepper.	15–20 minutes	Use in soups, salads, pasta dishes, and with roasted or mashed potatoes; flavor with garlic, olive oil, black pepper, basil, oregano, or herbes de Provence.
Mustard and turnip	1½–2 pounds	Wash to remove grit from leaves, and trim stems.	Steam or boil. Toss with olive oil, garlic, salt, and black pepper.	10–15 minutes	Cook with potatoes, mushrooms, and garlic; season greens with mustard, hot pepper, and cumin, and drizzle with olive oil.

Greens	Weight (4–6 Cooked Servings)	Prep	Cooking Methods	Approximate Cooking Times	Cooking Suggestions
Spinach	1½–2 pounds	Wash leaves thoroughly.	Young, tender spinach and mature spinach can both be steamed or eaten raw. Best sautéed in olive oil, garlic, salt, and black pepper.	3–5 minutes	Season cooked spinach with garlic and olive oil and use it in soups, with egg dishes, and in salads; season raw spinach with black pepper, any herbs, sea salt, and any dressing.
Stinging nettle	1½–2 pounds	Wash and strip leaves from stalks (stalks are too tough to eat).	Mild in flavor; cook by steaming. Toss with olive oil, garlic, salt, and black pepper.	3–5 minutes	Make nettle soup from stock and pureed nettle leaves; make nettle "pesto" with olive oil and pine nuts.

Greens Recipes

Braised Mustard Greens and Currants

Total Time: 25 minutes

Cut **2 bunches cleaned and trimmed mustard greens** into strips. Set aside. In a large skillet over medium heat, melt **2 tablespoons ghee or coconut oil.** Cook the mustard greens, **3 chopped cloves garlic,** and **1 teaspoon chopped fresh ginger** for 3 minutes. Add **1 cup vegetable stock or water.** Simmer for 15 minutes, or until the greens are tender. Remove from the heat and stir in ½ **cup black currants.**

MAKES 6 SERVINGS

Butternut Squash and Spinach Leaves

Total Time: 25 minutes

In a large skillet over medium-high heat, melt **2 tablespoons coconut oil** and **1 tablespoon ghee.** Cook **1 large red onion,** cut into thin wedges, ½ **teaspoon sea salt,** and ½ **tablespoon chopped fresh sage, or** ½ **teaspoon dried sage,** stirring occasionally, for 5 minutes, or until tender. Add **1 package (20 ounces) peeled and cubed butternut squash,** cover skillet, and cook, stirring occasionally, for 5 minutes, or until tender. Add **8 ounces baby spinach** and cook, stirring, for 1 minute or just until wilted. Transfer to a large platter. Sprinkle with **a handful of raisins** and/or **chopped walnuts.** Season with sea salt and **black pepper,** if desired.

MAKES 4 TO 6 SERVINGS

Carrots and Collards

Total Time: 30 minutes

1 pound collard greens chopped, and cut into strips. Set aside. In a large skillet over medium heat, melt **1 tablespoon coconut oil.** Cook **1 large chopped onion** and **2 sliced carrots** for 5 minutes, or until the onions are golden and the carrots are tender. Add the greens to the skillet. Cook, stirring occasionally, for 15 minutes. Sprinkle with a small **handful of chopped fresh parsley** and **1 to 2 tablespoons apple cider vinegar.**

MAKES 4 SERVINGS

Chard and Chickpea Stew

Total Time: 40 minutes

In a large pot over medium heat, melt **2 tablespoons coconut oil or ghee.** Cook **2 large chopped carrots, 1 chopped onion,** and **2 chopped ribs celery**, stirring occasionally, for 10 minutes, or until the vegetables are softened. Add **6 cups chicken stock** (preferably home-made) or water, **1 pound coarsely chopped Swiss chard, 1 can (15 ounces) rinsed and drained chickpeas, 1 tablespoon herbes de Provence,** and **½ teaspoon sea salt.** Simmer, stirring occasion-ally, for 20 minutes, or until the Swiss chard is tender.

MAKES 4 SERVINGS

Dandelion Frittata   Total Time: 35 minutes

Preheat the oven to 350°F. In a large bowl, beat **4 eggs and ½ cup plain soy milk or water.** Add **1 tablespoon chopped fresh basil.** In a large ovenproof skillet over medium heat, melt **1 tablespoon coconut oil.** Cook **1 small chopped onion, 4 ounces sliced mushrooms,** and **1 pound chopped dandelion greens,** stirring occasionally, for 5 minutes, or until softened. Pour the egg mixture over the onion mixture and cook, gently lifting the edges to let the uncooked portion flow underneath, for 5 minutes, or until the mixture just begins to set. Place the skillet in the oven and bake for 15 minutes, or until set.

MAKES 4 SERVINGS

Dandelion Greens with Toasted Mustard Seeds   Total Time: 15 minutes

Place a large dry skillet over medium heat. Toast **1 tablespoon yellow mustard seeds**, shaking the pan occasionally, for 1 to 2 minutes, or until the seeds are fragrant and just begin to pop. Transfer the seeds to a small bowl and set aside. In the same skillet, over medium-high heat, melt **2 tablespoons ghee.** Cook **1 pound trimmed and chopped dandelion greens**, stirring occasionally, for 5 minutes, or until tender. Remove from the heat and stir in the mustard seeds and **juice of 1 lemon**.

MAKES 4 SERVINGS

Lemony Beet Greens

Total Time: 15 minutes

Chop **1 pound beet greens,** into bite-size pieces. Set aside. In a large skillet over medium heat, melt **1 tablespoon ghee.** Cook **3 chopped cloves garlic** and the greens, stirring occasionally, for 10 minutes, or until the greens are tender. Sprinkle with ¼ **teaspoon black pepper** and the **juice of 1 lemon.**

MAKES 4 SERVINGS

Potato, Kale, and Leek Soup

Total Time: 55 minutes

In a large saucepan over medium heat, melt **2 tablespoons ghee or coconut oil.** Add **2 cleaned and chopped leeks, 1½ pounds peeled cubed organic potatoes,** and **1 cup water.** Simmer for 10 minutes, or until the potatoes are just tender. Add **5 cups vegetable stock** (preferably homemade) **or water** and **1 pound chopped kale.** Simmer, covered, stirring occasionally, for 30 minutes, or until the potatoes and kale are very tender. In a blender or with a hand blender, puree the soup. Season with sea salt and black pepper.

MAKES 4 SERVINGS

Salads

Salads make a great meal on a hot summer day, or a fresh side dish through all seasons. This go-to chart includes some simple, delicious meal options for all occasions.

Salad Greens	Average Weight (Servings)	Purchasing and Storing	Description	Cooking Suggestions
Arugula (also known as rocket; related to mustard greens)	1 bunch (2 servings)	Arugula tends to be gritty and should be soaked and washed if straight from the garden. Trim roots and use within 2 days. Leaves should be bright green.	Leaves are peppery; the larger the leaf, the more intense the flavor of this summer salad green.	Goes well with cooked pasta and can be used in pesto. Can be used by itself but a nice addition to any garden salad. Can be wilted and served with roasted chicken.
Escarole (related to the chicory family)	1 pound (8 servings)	Grown in spring to summer but available year-round. Leaves are leafy and bitter in taste. Separate leaves, cut ends, wash in cold water, and spin dry (unless adding to hot dishes). Keeps 3–5 days.	Packed with nutrition, this bitter green is high in fiber and vitamins.	Use in hot and cold dishes such as soups (Italian wedding or white bean) and grilled salads. It's good sautéed and served with a mild protein, such as cod or haddock.

Salad Greens	Average Weight (Servings)	Purchasing and Storing	Description	Cooking Suggestions
Mâche (also known as rapunzel, lamb's lettuce, and corn salad)	½ pound (4 servings)	Wash well, as it grows in sandy soil and tends to be gritty. Leaves should be dark green and look fresh.	Tender and earthy, this is a winter lettuce in most areas. (It originated in France.) Can be found in many spring mixes or can be mixed with other tender lettuces such as Boston or bibb, but wonderful on its own.	Goes well in salads, especially when combined with beets and walnuts or apples, oranges, and pine nuts. Use in potato salads and in omelets. Perfect with pumpkin seed oil, garlic, salt, and black pepper. Or very good with olive oil.
Romaine	½ pound romaine hearts (4 servings)	Look for organic heirloom cultivars when buying. Cut off ends, wash thoroughly under cold water, spin dry, and slice or chop. Will keep 5–7 days. (Leaves should be crisp when used.)	Romaine leaves are the mainstay of many classic salads because of their crispness. They're packed with nutrition but create a blank palate for other flavors in a dish.	Use in Caesar, Greek, and Mexican salads. (Try these classics without the cheese, or use soy cheese.) Great on sandwiches and can also replace the bread to make a low-calorie lettuce wrap sandwich filled with veggies.

Salad Recipes

Easy Arugula Salad with Egg

Total Time: 10 minutes

In a large bowl, whisk together **¼ cup olive oil mayonnaise, ¼ cup olive oil, 3 tablespoons white vinegar,** and **¼ teaspoon curry powder.** Add **8 cups baby arugula, 2 cups baby spinach, ¼ cup chopped fresh parsley,** and **2 chopped hard-cooked eggs.** Toss to coat well.

MAKES 6 SERVINGS

Romaine Salad

Total Time: 15 minutes

In a large bowl, whisk together **3 tablespoons olive oil, 2 tablespoons red wine vinegar,** and **2 tablespoons chopped fresh rosemary, thyme, oregano, or basil.** Add **1 large head chopped romaine lettuce, 1 small thinly sliced fennel bulb,** and a **handful of pine nuts.** Toss to coat well.

MAKES 4 SERVINGS

Mâche and Beet Salad

Total Time: 10 minutes

Arrange **8 ounces mâche (rapunzel) or baby arugula** on a large platter. Top with **4 cooked sliced beets, 4 sliced hard-cooked eggs,** and **1 sliced apple.** Drizzle with **1 to 2 tablespoons olive or pumpkin seed oil** and the **juice of 1 lemon**. Sprinkle with **2 tablespoons chopped fresh dill** and a **handful of pumpkin seeds.**

MAKES 4 SERVINGS

Spring Dandelion Salad

Total Time: 10 minutes

In a large bowl, combine **8 ounces chopped dandelion greens, ½ thinly sliced red onion,** and **1 pint sliced organic strawberries.** Drizzle with **1 to 2 tablespoons balsamic vinegar** and a **pinch each of sea salt** and **black pepper.** Toss to coat well. Sprinkle with a few **sliced almonds.**

MAKES 4 SERINGS

Vegetables

Go to the supermarket and determine which vegetables are the most affordable, look very fresh, and are organic. Then refer to this handy chart for easy, quick cooking methods.

Vegetable	Quantity for 4 Servings	Prep	Steam (Minutes)	Bake at 350°F (Minutes)	Cooking Suggestions
Artichokes	4 large or 8 small	Remove loose leaves. Cut off all but 1" of stem.	30–45	—	Great with green sauce (page 266).
Asparagus	1 pound	Break off woody stem where it easily snaps.	5–10	—	Steam and toss with olive oil and sesame seeds.
Beans, fava	2 pounds, unshelled	Remove beans from pods. If serving raw or lightly cooked, peel beans first; if cooking, peel afterward.	10–15	—	Good with savory.
Beans, shell (cranberry, lima)	2½ pounds unshelled or 1 pound shelled	Shell by snapping or cutting pod open and squeezing out beans.	15–25	—	Delicious with marjoram.
Beans, snap (green, wax)	1 pound	Snap off stem ends.	5–10	—	Good with savory.
Beets	1½ pounds	Scrub with a vegetable brush. Leave 1–2" of stems on. Slip off skins after cooking.	40–75	40–60	On first day serve as is; on second day serve as warm/cold salad.

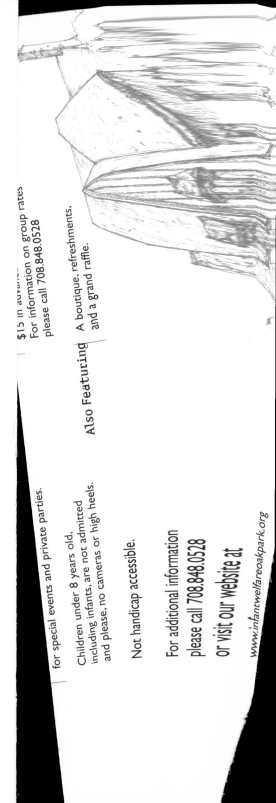

Vegetable	Quantity for 4 Servings	Prep	Steam (Minutes)	Bake at 350°F (Minutes)	Cooking Suggestions
Bok choy	1½ pounds	Leave baby bok choy whole. Separate larger heads from stalks. Cut off tough ends.	10–20	—	Sauté with olive oil, garlic, salt, and black pepper.
Broccoli	1½–2 pounds	Remove tough outer leaves and ends of stalks. Peel stalks if they're tough and cut into florets.	5–15	—	Sauté with garlic.
Broccolini	1½–2 pounds	Trim tough ends.	5–15	—	Sauté with garlic.
Broccoli rabe	1½–2 pounds	Trim tough ends.	5–15	—	Sauté with garlic.
Brussels sprouts	1½ pounds	Cut off stem ends and peel away any discolored leaves.	10–20	—	Sauté one large onion in coconut oil; simmer sprouts until done. Toss with melted ghee and caraway.
Cabbage, white	1 pound	Discard outer leaves. Halve or quarter.	9–12	—	Add nutmeg, salt, and black pepper.
Cabbage, napa	1 pound	Pull off any wilted leaves.	10–20	—	Prepare with red wine, jam, and olive oil.
Cabbage, red	1 pound	Discard outer leaves. Halve or quarter.	9–12	—	Serve with caraway.

Vegetable	Quantity for 4 Servings	Prep	Steam (Minutes)	Bake at 350°F (Minutes)	Cooking Suggestions
Carrots	1–2 pounds	Scrub with a vegetable brush. Peel thinly, if desired. Trim ends.	15–40	30–60	Prepare with ghee and parsley or dill.
Cauliflower	3–3½ pounds	Remove leaves.	5–25	—	Add nutmeg after cooking.
Corn	8 ears	Remove silk and husks, or remove silk only and soak in water to moisten husks.	10–15	—	Serve with herbed ghee.
Fennel	2 bulbs	Discard woody stalks. Save feathery fronds to use as an herb (and garnish). Halve or quarter bulb and cut away hard ends.	25–30	—	Serve with dill and its own leaves.
Greens, cooking, sturdy (collards, kale)	1½–2 pounds	Rinse thoroughly.	20–25	—	Prepare with olive oil, garlic, salt, and black pepper.
Greens, cooking, tender (beet, mustard, turnip)	1½–2 pounds	Rinse thoroughly. Remove thick stems, if desired.	5–10	—	Prepare with olive oil, garlic, salt, and black pepper.
Jerusalem artichokes	1 pound	Scrub with a vegetable brush. Peel thinly, if desired.	35	30–60	Good in stir-fries.
Kohlrabi	6–8 bulbs	Peel. Save greens for salads.	30–35	—	Best fresh, peeled—like an apple.

Vegetable	Quantity for 4 Servings	Prep	Steam (Minutes)	Bake at 350°F (Minutes)	Cooking Suggestions
Leeks	4 large	Cut off root ends. If using in pieces, cut up and rinse thoroughly. If using whole, split the leek up to where leaves look wilted and wash out soil caught between leaves.	10–20	—	Cook with 2 large onions in coconut oil; season with dill, salt, and black pepper.
Mushrooms, shiitake	1 pound	Wipe clean with a soft brush or damp cloth. Discard stems.	10	—	Sauté with garlic and olive oil.
Mushrooms, trumpet	8 ounces	Wipe clean with a soft brush or damp cloth. Discard stems.	5	15–20	Sauté with garlic and olive oil.
Okra	1 pound	Cut off stems.	20	—	Prepare with garlic, Italian seasoning, salt, and black pepper.
Onions	1½ pounds	Peel and cut off root ends.	—	50–60	Serve alone or with caraway.
Parsnips	1 pound	Scrub with a vegetable brush. Peel thinly, if desired. Trim ends.	35–40	35–40	Season with herbes de Provence.
Peas, edible pod (snow, sugar snaps)	1 pound	Snap off blossom ends. On sugar snaps, pull off string that runs down one side; on other peas, pull off strings from both sides.	5–10	—	Serve with dill, parsley, or ghee.

Vegetable	Quantity for 4 Servings	Prep	Steam (Minutes)	Bake at 350°F (Minutes)	Cooking Suggestions
Peas, green	2–3 pounds unshelled or 1 pound shelled	Split open pods and pop out peas.	10–20	—	Serve with dill, parsley, or ghee.
Potatoes, baking (organic only)	4 medium	Scrub with a vegetable brush and remove any eyes (sprouts). If baking whole, prick in several places to let steam escape.	—	45–60	Season with herbes de Provence.
Potatoes, waxy (organic only)	1½ pounds	Rinse. Cook unpeeled.	20–25	30–50	Serve with ghee and parsley.
Pumpkin	2–3 pounds	Halve and remove stringy pulp and seeds. (Save seeds for roasting.)	25–30	60	Serve with ghee, salt, and black pepper.
Rutabaga (Swedes, yellow turnips)	1–2 pounds	Peel if waxed.	35–40	—	Season with olive oil, salt, and black pepper.
Salsify (oyster plants)	1–1½ pounds	Cut off tops. Peel thinly if desired.	10	35–40	Prepare with ghee and thyme.
Spinach	1½–2 pounds	Rinse thoroughly.	3–5	—	Prepare with olive oil, garlic, salt, and black pepper.

Vegetable	Quantity for 4 Servings	Prep	Steam (Minutes)	Bake at 350°F (Minutes)	Cooking Suggestions
Squash, spaghetti	3–4 pounds	Halve and seed. Add a little water to the baking pan, cover with foil, and steam-bake, cut sides down.	—	60	Add ghee or olive oil *after* baking.
Squash, summer	2–3 pounds	Cut off stems and blossom ends.	15–20	30–60	Boil with some olive oil. Add salt and black pepper after cooking.
Squash, winter	2–3 pounds	Peel and halve. Remove seeds after baking.	25–30	60	Season with olive oil, salt, and black pepper after cooking.
Sweet potatoes	1–2 pounds	Scrub well. Peel if cutting up.	—	30–50	Season with rosemary.
Swiss chard	1½–2 pounds	Rinse thoroughly. Trim off any split or bruised ends from the ribs.	5–10	—	Prepare with olive oil, garlic, salt, and black pepper.
Turnips	1–2 pounds	Cut off roots and greens (save greens); scrub and peel thinly, if desired.	15–25	—	Season with marjoram and caraway.

Vegetable Recipes

Asian Slaw

Total Time: 15 minutes + chilling time

In a large bowl, whisk together **½ cup olive oil mayonnaise, ¼ cup rice vinegar, 1 teaspoon sesame seeds,** and **½ teaspoon toasted sesame oil.** Add **4 cups thinly sliced cabbage, 2 large shredded carrots, ¼ cup chopped fresh cilantro, 2 minced cloves garlic,** and **1 teaspoon minced fresh ginger.** Toss to coat well. Refrigerate for 1 hour before serving.

MAKES 4 TO 6 SERVINGS

Broccoli and Spaghetti

Total Time: 25 minutes

Prepare **1 medium spaghetti squash** according to chart (page 223). Cut **1 bunch broccoli** into small florets and add to the pasta during the last 3 minutes of cooking time. In the pasta cooking pot over medium heat, melt **1 tablespoon coconut oil.** Cook **2 chopped cloves garlic,** stirring frequently, for 2 minutes, or until golden. Add **1 cup canned unsweetened coconut milk** and **½ teaspoon ground turmeric.** Stir in the spaghetti squash and broccoli. Cook, tossing to coat well, for 1 minute, or until heated through.

MAKES 4 TO 6 SERVINGS

Breakfast Beans

Total Time: 10 minutes

In a small saucepan over medium heat, warm **1 to 2 tablespoons olive oil.** Cook **1 tablespoon dried herbs such as savory, dill, parsley, cilantro, or tarragon.** Add **1 can (14.5 ounces) rinsed and drained organic beans.** Cook, stirring, for 3 minutes, or until heated through. Sprinkle with a **pinch of sea salt or a pinch of pepper.**

MAKES 1 TO 2 SERVINGS

Celeriac Salad

Total Time: 35 minutes

Boil **1 pound celeriac** (also known as celery root) in a large pot of lightly salted water until tender. Drain. Peel and cube. Transfer to a large bowl. Add **1 small finely chopped red onion, 4 tablespoons olive oil, 1 teaspoon apple cider vinegar,** and **sea salt and black pepper.** Stir in a **handful of chopped fresh dill, tarragon, or chives** and toss to coat well.

MAKES 4 SERVINGS

Variation:

- *Use red or golden beets in place of celeriac.*

Cold Green Bean Salad
Total Time: 10 minutes + chilling time

Place a steamer basket in a large pot with 2" of water. Bring to a boil over high heat. Steam **1 pound trimmed green beans** in the basket for 3 minutes, or until tender-crisp. Cover and refrigerate for 30 minutes, or until chilled. Meanwhile, in a large bowl, whisk together **2 tablespoons olive oil, 2 tablespoons lemon juice,** and **½ teaspoon chopped fresh parsley, chives, thyme, or tarragon.** Add the green beans, **1 teaspoon sesame seeds or white chia seeds,** and a **pinch of sea salt.** Toss to coat well.

MAKES 4 SERVINGS

Cucumber Salad
Total Time: 10 minutes

In a large bowl, combine **1 large thinly sliced organic cucumber, ½ cup thinly sliced red onion, 1 or 2 tablespoons chopped fresh dill or 1 or 2 teaspoons dried dillweed, 1 tablespoon white vinegar,** and **sea salt** and **black pepper.** Fold in **¼ to ½ cup Whipped Coconut Cream** (page 269), just enough to moisten the cucumbers without them getting too watery, and toss to coat well.

MAKES 4 SERVINGS

Variations:

• *Use sliced Belgian endive, spinach leaves, or romaine lettuce in place of the cucumber.*

• *For those lazy summer evenings, turn this salad into a main dish meal using the best of summer's produce. Add some organic corn, summer squash, carrots, or cooked broccoli.*

• *You may also add, sparingly though, a little leftover cooked quinoa or brown rice, or a bit of cooked chicken, turkey, or fish.*

Curried Spaghetti Squash

Total Time: 1 hour 10 minutes

Preheat the oven to 350°F. Cut **1 medium spaghetti squash** in half lengthwise. Brush the cut sides with **2 teaspoons olive oil.** Place both halves, cut sides down, on a small baking sheet. With a fork, pierce the squash halves in several places. Roast for 45 minutes, or until very tender when pierced with a fork. Let cool for 10 minutes, then scoop out the seeds. Meanwhile, in a large skillet over medium-high heat, melt **1 tablespoon ghee** and **1 tablespoon coconut oil.** Cook **2 chopped cloves garlic** and **2 teaspoons chopped fresh ginger** for 3 minutes, or until softened. With a fork, scrape the spaghetti-like strands of squash into the skillet. Add **1 cup unsweetened coconut milk, 1 teaspoon curry powder, ½ teaspoon ground cinnamon,** and **sea salt** and **black pepper.** Simmer, stirring gently, for 5 minutes, or until heated through. Serve sprinkled with a **handful of chopped fresh cilantro.**

MAKES 6 SERVINGS

Herbal Soup

Total Time: 50 minutes

Place **1 teaspoon whole peppercorns** in a metal tea ball or in a piece of cheesecloth and tie it closed with string. In a large skillet, heat **2 tablespoons olive oil** over medium-high heat. Add **3 large chopped onions, 6 to 8 peeled, halved cloves garlic,** and **a handful of dried herbs such as marjoram, rosemary, or thyme.** Cook, stirring occasionally, for 5 minutes, or until the onions and garlic are lightly browned and tender. Remove from heat. Fill a large pot with **8 cups water** and bring to a boil over high heat. Add the onion mixture, **4 cups cubed root vegetables such as parsnips or turnips,** the whole peppercorns in the tea ball or cheesecloth, and **1 teaspoon herbal salt (preferably Herbamare*)** and bring to a boil. Reduce the heat and simmer, stirring occasionally, for 20 minutes, or until the vegetables are tender. Add ½ **pound trimmed green beans, cut into 1" pieces,** or **2 large zucchini or yellow squash, cut into 1" pieces.** Return to a boil and cook for 5 minutes, stirring occasionally. Add **1 bunch greens such as spinach, dandelion, chard, or kale** and simmer for 3 minutes, or until the vegetables are tender. Remove from the heat and stir in ¼ **cup chopped fresh basil or parsley.** Remove peppercorns. Season with **sea salt** and **ground black pepper** to taste.

A fresh soup like this is different every time because the available vegetables and herbs change throughout the seasons.

MAKES 10 TO 12 SERVINGS

*Herbamare is a combination of organic herbs, vegetables, and sea salt. You can find it in the spice section of most supermarkets or in health food stores.

Variations:

• *Use any vegetables you have on hand, such as celeriac, white cabbage, savoy cabbage, carrots, kale, green beans, chard, dandelion greens, leeks, mushrooms, cauliflower, peppers, summer squash, tomatoes, or broccoli.*

• *Add spices—anything goes, from caraway to basil to curry to parsley and more. Be inventive!*

Kohlrabi Salad

Total Time: 15 minutes

In a large bowl, combine **2 medium kohlrabi, peeled and cut into 1 piece (3") daikon, peeled and cut into thin slices, 1 small finely chopped red onion, ¼ cup chopped fresh mint, 2 tablespoons rice wine vinegar, 2 tablespoons olive oil,** and **sea salt** and **black pepper.** Toss to mix well. If you prefer a sweeter salad, you may add a bit of **stevia.**

MAKES 4 TO 6 SERVINGS

Egg Salad

Total Time: 10 minutes

Coarsely chop **8 hard-cooked eggs** and transfer to a large bowl. Add **1 small finely chopped onion, 1 finely chopped rib celery, ¼ cup mayonnaise, 2 teaspoons chopped fresh herbs such as tarragon, dill, chives, basil, or parsley (or ½ teaspoon dried herbs), 1 heaping teaspoon Dijon mustard,** and a **pinch each of sea salt** and **black pepper.** Toss to mix well.

MAKES 4 SERVINGS

Variation:

- *Use leftover cooked chicken or canned tuna in place of the eggs.*

Leek and Onion Frittata

Total Time: 40 minutes

Preheat the oven to 400°F. In a large bowl, beat **8 eggs** with **¼ cup warm water, ¼ cup fresh chopped herbs (such as parsley, oregano, and thyme),** and a **pinch each of sea salt** and **black pepper.** In a large ovenproof skillet over medium-high heat, melt **1 tablespoon ghee** and **1 tablespoon olive oil.** Cook **2 chopped onions** and **2 cleaned sliced leeks,** stirring occasionally, for 10 minutes, or until golden. Pour the egg mixture over the onion mixture and cook, gently lifting the edges to let the uncooked portion flow underneath, for 5 minutes, or until the mixture just begins to set. Place the skillet in the oven and bake for 15 minutes, or until a knife inserted in the center comes out clean.

MAKES 4 SERVINGS

Marinated Vegetables

Total Time: 20 minutes + marinating and standing time

In a large bowl, whisk together **1 cup olive oil, ½ cup white wine or champagne vinegar, 1 teaspoon crushed fennel seeds or 1 teaspoon dried oregano or basil,** a **pinch of ground red pepper,** and a **pinch of sea salt and pepper** until blended. Add **3 cups cauliflower florets, 2 cups halved Brussels sprouts, 1 large thinly sliced red onion,** and **2 sliced carrots.** Toss to mix well. Cover and marinate in the refrigerator for at least 2 hours or overnight. Let the vegetables stand for 20 minutes at room temperature before serving.

MAKES 4 TO 6 SERVINGS

Mashed Neeps

Total Time: 40 minutes

In a large saucepan, combine **2 pounds peeled cubed parsnips, 1 large peeled cubed rutabaga,** and **2 large peeled cubed organic Yukon Gold potatoes** with enough cold water to cover by 2". Bring to a boil over high heat. Reduce the heat to medium-low, cover, and simmer for 20 minutes, or until the vegetables are tender. Drain and return to the pot. Add ⅓ **cup melted ghee** and ½ **cup vegetable stock** and mash with a potato masher until smooth. Season with **sea salt** and **black pepper.**

MAKES 4 TO 6 SERVINGS

Organic Corn on the Cob with Herbed Ghee

Prepare **8 ears organic corn** according to chart on page 220. Meanwhile, prepare one of the Herbed Ghee recipes below to serve with the corn.

Herbed Ghee

Total Time: 10 minutes

For a Latin flair, add **2 tablespoons lime juice, 1 tablespoon chopped fresh cilantro, 1 tablespoon chopped fresh parsley,** and a **pinch each of sea salt** and **black pepper** to **1 cup melted ghee.**

For Italian flavors, add **2 tablespoons chopped fresh basil, 2 teaspoons lemon juice, 1 teaspoon dried oregano,** and a **pinch each of sea salt** and **black pepper** to **1 cup melted ghee.**

MAKES 8 SERVINGS

Poached Egg in Onion Hash

Total Time: 25 minutes

In a small skillet over medium heat, melt **1 tablespoon coconut oil.** Add **2 thinly sliced onions and a pinch of sea salt** and **black pepper.** Cook, stirring occasionally, for 8 minutes, or until golden. With a spoon, make a "nest" in the center of the onions. Crack **1 egg** on the rim of the skillet and gently slide it into the nest without breaking the yolk. Reduce the heat to low, cover, and cook for 5 minutes, or until the egg white is firm but the yolk is still soft.

MAKES 1 SERVING

Rice and Peas

Total Time: 50 minutes

In a large saucepan over medium-high heat, melt **2 tablespoons ghee.** Cook **1 chopped onion**, stirring occasionally, for 5 minutes, or until softened. Add **2 cups water, 1 cup vegetable stock or water,** and **1 cup uncooked brown rice.** Bring to a boil. Reduce the heat to low, cover, and simmer for 30 minutes. Stir in **3 cups fresh peas** and cook for 5 minutes, or until the liquid is absorbed, the rice and peas are tender. Fluff the rice mixture with a fork and stir in **2 tablespoons chopped fresh parsley** and **1 teaspoon grated lemon peel.**

MAKES 4 SERVINGS

Roasted Baby Potatoes

Total Time: 30 minutes

In a large skillet over medium heat, melt **1 to 2 tablespoons coconut oil.** Sauté **1 pound small whole organic baby potatoes,** covered, turning the potatoes occasionally, for 20 minutes, or until the potatoes are tender and lightly browned. Stir in **1 tablespoon olive oil, 1 tablespoon chopped fresh rosemary or 1 teaspoon dried rosemary,** and a **pinch of sea salt** and **black pepper.**

MAKES 4 SERVINGS

Variations:

- *Use your choice of herbs, fresh or dried. Marjoram is delicious.*
- *Chopped onions and garlic can also be used to round out this dish. Add 1 small sliced onion and 2 chopped cloves garlic with the potatoes.*
- *Larger potatoes, cut into ½" slices, may be used instead of smaller potatoes. Whatever the size, be sure to always use organic potatoes.*

Skillet Baby Carrots and Snap Peas

Total Time: 15 minutes

In a large skillet over medium-high heat, melt **2 tablespoons ghee** with **2 chopped cloves garlic** and **1 teaspoon chopped fresh ginger.** Cook, stirring constantly, for 1 minute, or until fragrant. Stir in **2 cups baby carrots** and **2 cups snap peas or snow peas** and cook for 5 minutes, or until tender-crisp. Sprinkle with **sliced almonds, chopped fresh parsley,** and **grated lemon peel.**

MAKES 4 SERVINGS

Vegetable Stir-Fry

Total Time: 30 minutes

In a medium bowl, soak **1 ounce dried shiitake mushrooms** in ¾ **cup water** for 15 minutes. Meanwhile, in a large skillet or wok over medium-high heat, heat 2 **tablespoons coconut oil.** Add **2 chopped cloves garlic** and **1 teaspoon grated ginger** and cook for 1 minute. Add **2 large carrots, cut into thick slices,** and **1 thinly sliced red bell pepper** and cook, stirring constantly, for 5 minutes, or until golden and tender-crisp. Add the soaked mushrooms with their liquid and **4 ounces sliced wild mushrooms** to the skillet. Cook for 4 minutes, or until golden and softened. Add **2 teaspoons toasted sesame oil** and **2 tablespoons tamari soy sauce** and stir to coat vegetables. Reduce the heat to medium. Cover and cook for 1 minute. Remove from heat and garnish with **2 thinly sliced scallions.**

MAKES 2 SERVINGS

White Beans and Rabe

Total Time: 35 minutes

Place a steamer basket in a large saucepot with 2" of water. Bring to a boil over high heat. Cook **1 bunch broccoli rabe,** trimmed and tough stems removed, in the basket for 2 minutes, or until tender, and drain. Meanwhile, in a large skillet over medium-high heat, heat **1 tablespoon olive oil.** Cook **4 minced cloves garlic,** stirring constantly, for 1 minute, or until fragrant. Add **2 cups sliced shiitake and/or trumpet mushrooms** and ½ **cup vegetable stock** (preferably homemade) **or water,** and bring to a simmer. Cook over medium-high heat, stirring occasionally, for 15 minutes, or until the mushrooms are tender and the liquid is evaporated. Stir in the broccoli rabe and **1 can (15 ounces) rinsed and drained white beans.** Cook, stirring occasionally, for 2 minutes, or until heated through. Season with **sea salt** and **black pepper.**

MAKES 4 SERVINGS

Grains

If you purchase grains with their bran layers intact—whole grain barley, kamut, rye, spelt, triticale, and wheat—try soaking them overnight to shorten your cooking time by at least an hour. Bring to a boil, cover with a lid, and then simmer on low. The grain is done when all the water is soaked up.

1 Cup Dry Grain	Water (cups)	Approximate Cooking Time	Cooked Yield (cups)
Amaranth	2	20–25 minutes	2½
Barley, pearled	3	55 minutes	3
Buckwheat groats	2	20–25 minutes	2½
Cornmeal	4	25 minutes	3
Farro, semipearled	3	30 minutes	3
Farro, unhulled	3	2 hours	3⅔
Kamut	3	2 hours	2⅔
Kasha (toasted buckwheat)	2	15–20 minutes	3
Millet	3	45 minutes	3½
Oats, rolled	3	15 minutes	3½
Oats, steel-cut	3	30–40 minutes	3½
Quinoa	2	12–15 minutes	3½
Rice, black	2	30 minutes	3
Rice, brown	2	35–45 minutes	3
Rice, red	2	20 minutes	3
Rice, white	2	20 minutes	3
Rice, wild	3	1 hour	4
Rye berries	4	1 hour	2⅔
Sorghum	3	45 minutes	3½
Spelt	3	2 hours	2⅔
Triticale	4	1 hour	2½

Grain Recipes

Lentil Soup

Total Time: 55 minutes

In a large saucepan over medium-high heat, heat **2 tablespoons olive oil.** Cook **2 chopped carrots, 2 chopped ribs celery,** and **2 chopped cloves garlic,** stirring occasionally, for 4 minutes, or until softened. Add **6 cups vegetable stock, ½ cup brown lentils,** and **1 to 2 teaspoons ground cumin.** Bring to a boil. Reduce the heat to low, cover, and simmer for 20 minutes, or just until the lentils are tender. Stir in **1 to 2 chopped fresh tomatoes** and cook over medium-high heat, stirring occasionally, for 5 minutes, or until the tomatoes are softened. Add **1 container (5 ounces) baby spinach or 1 small bunch chopped Swiss chard.** Cook the spinach, stirring occasionally, for 3 minutes, or just until wilted. If using Swiss chard, cook for 6 minutes, or just until tender. Season with **sea salt** and **black pepper.**

MAKES 4 SERVINGS

Fruity Quinoa

Total Time: 30 minutes

In a large saucepan, bring **1 cup water, ½ cup quinoa, 1 tablespoon ghee,** and **1 teaspoon ground cinnamon** to a boil over high heat. Reduce the heat to medium, cover, and simmer for 15 minutes, or just until the bulgur is tender and the liquid is absorbed. Remove from the heat and stir in **1 cup berries.**

MAKES 4 SERVINGS

Quinoa Onion Pilaf

Total Time: 45 minutes

In a large skillet over medium heat, melt **2 tablespoons coconut oil.** Cook **1 large chopped red or yellow onion** for 5 minutes, or just until softened. Add **3 minced cloves garlic** and cook for 1 minute, stirring, or until fragrant. Stir in **2 cups vegetable stock or water** and **1 cup quinoa,** and bring to a boil. Reduce the heat to low, cover, and simmer for 20 minutes, or until the quinoa is tender and the liquid is absorbed. Remove from the heat. Stir in a **small handful of chopped fresh cilantro** and sprinkle with **2 thinly sliced scallions.**

MAKES 4 SERVINGS

Meats

Refer to the cooking charts below for simple, straightforward instructions on days when you're adding meat to your meals. Stick with organic, grass-fed meat, which is less inflammatory than feedlot meat.

Cooking Times for Meat: Roasting

The times given below will produce meat cooked to 135°F (medium-rare). If you like your meat rarer or more well-done, adjust times accordingly. Keep in mind that meat temperatures will rise about 5°F while sitting. An instant-read thermometer is a good and inexpensive investment. Meats are delicious rubbed with fresh or dried herbs before roasting. Beef works well with thyme, rosemary, and garlic. Lamb is delicious with mint and parsley or curry. Season pork with cinnamon, ginger, and cloves.

Cut of Meat	Approximate Cooking Time per Pound at 350°F (Minutes)
Beef, bottom round	17–18
Beef, eye round	20–22
Beef, rib roast	15–18
Beef, ribs	35–45
Beef, rump roast	15–17
Beef, sirloin, tri-tip	12–15
Beef, tenderloin	12–15
Lamb, chops	25–30
Lamb, crown roast	25–30
Lamb, leg, bone-in	17–18
Lamb, leg, boneless	15–17
Lamb, rib roast "rack"	10–12
Pork, loin, bone-in	25–30
Pork, loin, boneless	17–18
Pork, rib roast	25–30
Pork, ribs	35–45
Pork, tenderloin	15–16

Cooking Times for Meat: Broiling

The cooking times below are based on broiling or grilling 4 to 6 inches from the heat source. Broilers and grills vary in heat intensity, so as a rule of thumb, check the meat a few minutes before the time indicated to avoid overcooking. Be sure to keep broiled meats to a minimum to avoid ingestion of AGEs.

Meat	Cut	Thickness (Inches)	Approximate Cooking Time for Rare (Minutes)	Approximate Cooking Time for Medium (Minutes)	Approximate Cooking Time for Well-Done (Minutes)
Beef	Chuck, boneless	1	7	9	14
	Chuck, with bone	1	8	10	15
	Cubes for kebabs	1	6–8	8–9	12
	Ground, burger	1	6	10	14
	Steak, flank	1	8	10	14
	Steaks: club, filet mignon, porterhouse, rib, sirloin, T-bone	1	6	8	12–15
Lamb	Boneless leg, butterflied	4	30	40	55
	Chops, loin, rib, shoulder	1	7–8	9–10	12
	Cubes for kebabs	1	6–7	8–9	12
	Ground, burger	1	6	10	14
Pork	Chops	1	—	9–10	12
	Cubes for kebabs	1	—	8–9	12

Meat and Poultry Recipes

Beef

Flank Steak with Roasted Vegetables

Total Time: 55 minutes

Preheat the oven to 350°F. In a large, shallow roasting pan, combine **2 cups broccoli florets, 2 cups cubed winter or summer squash, 1 cup sliced carrots,** and **3 tablespoons coconut oil.** Sprinkle with **sea salt** and **black pepper,** and toss to coat well. Roast, stirring occasionally, for 20 minutes, or just until the vegetables are tender. Meanwhile, sprinkle a **1-pound flank steak** with **2 tablespoons lime juice.** In a large skillet over medium-high heat, heat **1 tablespoon coconut oil.** Cook the steak for 8 minutes, turning once, or until an instant-read thermometer inserted in the center registers 145°F for medium-rare. Transfer the steak to a cutting board and let stand for 5 minutes before thinly slicing across the grain. Serve the steak with the vegetables.

MAKES 4 SERVINGS

Quick Chili

Total Time: 55 minutes

In a large saucepan over medium-high heat, cook **1 pound 95% lean ground beef,** breaking it up with a spoon, for 3 minutes, until just cooked. Add **1 chopped onion, 1 medium chopped summer or winter squash, 1 bulb minced cloves garlic,** and **1 teaspoon ground cumin.** Cook for 8 minutes, stirring occasionally, or until the onion is softened. Stir in **3½ cups vegetable stock or water,** and **1 can (15 ounces) rinsed and drained red or black beans.** Bring to a boil. Reduce the heat to medium-low, cover, and simmer, stirring occasionally, for 15 minutes, or until the flavors are blended. Sprinkle with a **handful of thinly sliced scallions or chives** before serving.

MAKES 4 SERVINGS

Lamb

Lamb Curry

Total Time: 1 hour 15 minutes

In a large skillet over medium-high heat, melt **1 tablespoon coconut oil.** Cook **1 pound cubed boneless lean lamb** for 5 minutes. Transfer to a plate. Melt **1 tablespoon coconut oil** in the same skillet over medium heat. Cook **2 chopped onions** and **3 chopped cloves garlic,** stirring occasionally, for 8 minutes, or until the onions are very tender. Add **1 tablespoon curry powder, ½ teaspoon ground cinnamon,** and **¼ teaspoon ground cardamom** and cook for 30 seconds, or until fragrant. Return the lamb to the skillet along with **1 cup vegetable stock or water** and **1 cup fresh canned pineapple or 1 cup cubed apples.** Bring to a boil. Reduce the heat to low, cover, and simmer for 30 minutes. Add **2 cups cubed parsnips** and cook, stirring occasionally, for 15 minutes, or until the **parsnips** are tender. Stir in **1 cup fresh or frozen peas** and cook for 5 minutes, or until tender. Serve over **brown rice or quinoa.**

MAKES 4 SERVINGS

Lean Lamb Burgers

Total Time: 15 minutes

In a large bowl, mix together **1 pound lean ground lamb, 1 small finely chopped onion, 1 egg, 1 tablespoon chopped fresh mint (or 1 tablespoon dried Italian seasoning),** and **1 to 2 minced cloves garlic.** Form the mixture into 4 patties. In a large skillet over medium heat, melt **1 tablespoon coconut oil.** Cook the burgers for 8 minutes, turning once, or until an instant-read thermometer inserted in the center of a burger registers 165°F.

MAKES 4 SERVINGS

Herbed Lamb Chops

Total Time: 15 minutes

In a small bowl, combine **3 tablespoons lemon juice, 3 minced cloves garlic,** and **1 teaspoon chopped fresh thyme, mint, or rosemary.** Mix well. Brush both sides of **4 bone-in lamb shoulder chops (5 ounces each)** with the lemon mixture. In a large skillet over medium-high heat, heat **1 tablespoon olive oil.** Cook the chops for 6 minutes, turning once, or until a thermometer inserted in the center registers 145°F for medium-rare. Serve with **sautéed baby spinach or kale.**

MAKES 4 SERVINGS

Leg of Lamb

Total Time: 2 hours 15 minutes

Preheat the oven to 350°F. In a Dutch oven or clay pot over medium-high heat, heat **1 tablespoon olive oil.** Cook 1 **boneless leg of lamb (3½ to 4 pounds)** for 5 minutes, turning occasionally. With tongs, transfer to a large plate. Add **3 large chopped onions, 2 thinly sliced carrots, 1 package (8 ounces) sliced cremini mushrooms,** and **2 large peeled cubed parsnips** and cook, stirring occasionally, for 6 minutes, or until softened. Add **3 cups dry red wine, 1 teaspoon herbal salt** (preferably Herbamare*), **1 teaspoon whole black peppercorns** (in a tea ball or wrapped and tied in cheesecloth), and a **small handful of rosemary or herbes de Provence.** Place in the oven and bake for 2 hours, or until the lamb is fork-tender. Remove the whole peppercorns before serving.

MAKES 8 SERVINGS

*Herbamare is a combination of organic herbs, vegetables, and sea salt. You can find it in the spice section of most supermarkets or in health food stores.

Variations:

- *Use different vegetables like leeks, zucchini, or summer squash.*
- *Incorporate fresh herbs from the garden or dried herb mixtures.*

Pork

Slow Cooker Pork and Vegetables

Total Time: 2½ to 3 hours on high, or 4½ to 5 hours on low

Place **2 large sliced onions** in a 5- to 6-quart slow cooker. In a large skillet over medium-high heat, warm **1 tablespoon olive oil**. Sprinkle **1 pound boneless pork tenderloin** with ½ **teaspoon kosher salt,** ¼ **teaspoon ground black pepper,** and ¼ **teaspoon ground cumin.** Place the pork on top of the onions. Scatter **3 medium chopped carrots** and **8 ounces sliced mushrooms** around the pork. Pour **1 cup vegetable stock** and **2 tablespoons apple cider vinegar** over the pork. Cover and cook for 2 to 3 hours on high or 4 to 5 hours on low. About 40 minutes before the cooking time is up, add **2 large sliced Granny Smith apples** to the slow cooker. Cover and cook for 40 minutes, or until the pork is fork-tender.

MAKES 6 SERVINGS

Pork and Broccoli Stir-Fry

Total Time: 30 minutes

Cut a **1 pound pork tenderloin** into 1" pieces. Sprinkle with **½ teaspoon kosher salt** and **¼ teaspoon ground black pepper.** In a large skillet over medium-high heat, melt **2 tablespoons coconut oil.** Cook the pork for 5 minutes, turning. Add **2 minced cloves garlic** and **1 teaspoon chopped fresh ginger** and cook for 1 minute, or until fragrant. Add **1 cup broccoli florets** and **2 tablespoons water** and cover and cook for 2 minutes, or until broccoli is tender crisp. Add **2 cups snow peas, 1 cup broccoli florets,** and **1 can (8 ounces) unsweetened pineapple chunks with juice.** Bring to a boil. Reduce the heat and simmer for 3 minutes, stirring occasionally, or until the sauce thickens slightly and the vegetables are tender-crisp. Serve over **brown rice.**

MAKES 4 SERVINGS

Poultry

Poultry should be roasted at low temperatures (325° to 350°F) or high (400°F). When properly cooked and ready to eat, the breast meat should register 160° to 165°F on an instant-read thermometer. The thigh needs to cook to 170° to 175°F. Remember that all poulty needs to be organic and free-range. Before roasting a duck, pierce skin all over, every ½ inch. While roasting, carefully remove the duck and pierce skin every hour. The breast meat should register 165°F on an instant-read thermometer.

Poultry		Weight (pounds)	Oven Temperature (°F)	Approximate Roasting Time
Capon		8–10	400	1 hour 40 minutes
Chicken, whole	Broiler/fryer	3–5	400	1 hour
	Stuffer/roaster	6–8	400	1 hour 25 minutes
Cornish hen		1–2	400	30–40 minutes
Duck, whole		5–7	300	3–4 hours
Goose		10–12	325	3 hours
Turkey	Breast, bone-in, half	3–5	325	1 hour 15 minutes
	Breast, bone-in, whole	5–7	325	2 hours 15 minutes
	Whole	8–12	350	2 hours 45 minutes
		12–14	350	3 hours 30 minutes
		14–18	350	3 hours 45 minutes
		20–24	325	5 hours

Poultry Recipes
Easy Broiled Chicken with Herbs

Total Time: 25 minutes

Line a broiler-pan rack with foil. Brush the foil with olive oil and preheat the broiler.

Brush **4 boneless, skinless chicken breasts or boneless, skinless chicken thighs (4 to 6 ounces each)** with **2 tablespoons melted ghee.** Sprinkle the chicken with **1 teaspoon dried rosemary, thyme, or herbes de Provence.** Place the chicken on the broiler-pan rack and broil 8" from the heat source for 8 minutes, turning once, for breasts, or for 15 minutes, turning once, for thighs, or until an instant-read thermometer inserted in the thickest portion registers 165°F and the juices run clear.

MAKES 4 SERVINGS

Herbed Turkey Burgers

Total Time: 20 minutes

In a large bowl, mix together **1 pound lean ground organic turkey, 1 finely chopped onion,** a **handful of chopped fresh basil or 2 teaspoons dried Italian seasoning, 1 egg, 5 minced cloves garlic, 1 teaspoon olive oil, a pinch of sea salt** and **½ teaspoon ground black pepper.** Form the mixture into 8 patties.

In a large skillet over medium-high heat, melt **1 tablespoon coconut oil.** Cook the burgers for 8 minutes, turning once, or until an instant-read thermometer inserted in the center registers 165°F and the meat is no longer pink. Serve with cooked **brown rice** and **steamed vegetables.** Burgers can also be frozen before cooking. This is a good dish to prepare on a weekend for the following week.

Makes 8 servings

Variations:

• *Use ground beef, lamb, or chicken in place of the ground turkey.*

• *Incorporate different herbs (fresh or dried) to see which tastes you prefer.*

Fish and Shellfish

In general, fish is best when prepared and cooked quickly and simply, making it part of an ideal weeknight meal. See the chart below for easy cooking instructions. Fish should be cooked until opaque. Fillets and steaks should flake easily with a fork. Add 5 to 10 minutes cook time for frozen fish. And remember to avoid farmed fish.

Fish	Cooking Methods	Baking (350°F)
Fillets (salmon, cod, hake, haddock, snapper, halibut, grouper, bluefish, mackerel)	Coat with oil (olive or coconut) and bake, steam, or cook in a skillet.	10 minutes for each inch of thickness, until opaque and flakes easily
Whole fish (red snapper, branzino, bass, bluefish, grouper, mackerel, herring, smelt)	Coat with oil (olive or coconut) and stuff with lemon slices and herbs. Bake or steam.	20–30 minutes, depending on the thickness of fish (10 minutes per inch)
Lobster tails	Steam or bake; serve drizzled with melted ghee.	20–25 minutes
Whole lobster	Steam or bake. Serve with melted ghee.	18–20 minutes, turning once
Mussels	Steam; serve with melted ghee, garlic, and thyme.	—
Shrimp (wild-caught only)	Steam, bake, or cook on skillet with oil and garlic.	15–20 minutes
Squid, sliced	Cook in a skillet or bake coated with olive oil, garlic, and oregano or rosemary.	10–15 minutes

Fish Recipes

Broiled Trout

Total Time: 15 minutes

Brush a broiler-pan rack with olive oil. Preheat the broiler. In a small bowl, combine **2 tablespoons olive oil mayonnaise, 1 tablespoon chopped fresh tarragon or dill, 1 teaspoon lemon juice,** and **1 minced clove garlic** until well blended. Evenly brush the mayonnaise mixture on **4 trout fillets (4 ounces each).** Place the fillets on the broiler-pan rack and broil on low 4" from the heat source for 3 minutes, or until the fish flakes easily. Do not turn. Sprinkle the fillets with sliced almonds and serve.

MAKES 4 SERVINGS

Cod and Shrimp Stew

Total Time: 25 minutes

In a large saucepan over medium-high heat, heat **2 tablespoons olive oil.** Cook **1 chopped bulb garlic,** and **¼ teaspoon red-pepper flakes,** stirring occasionally, for 2 minutes, or until softened. Stir in **2 cans (14.5 ounces each) diced tomatoes** and cook for 5 minutes. Add **1 pound peeled and deveined large shrimp** and **1 pound cod fillet, cut into 2" pieces.** Bring to a simmer. Reduce the heat to low, cover, and simmer for 5 minutes, or until the shrimp and cod are just opaque. Serve sprinkled with **chopped fresh cilantro or parsley.**

MAKES 4 SERVINGS

Grilled Miso-Glazed Salmon

Total Time: 25 minutes

Preheat the grill to medium. Coat an 11" x 7" shallow baking pan with olive oil. In a small bowl, combine **2 tablespoons red miso paste, 1 tablespoon rice wine vinegar, 1 teaspoon minced fresh ginger, 1 teaspoon gluten-free tamari sauce,** and a **pinch of ground black pepper** until well blended. Rub all over **4 salmon fillets (6 ounces each).** Place the fillets in the pan. Place the pan over direct heat and grill, covered, for 15 minutes, or until the salmon is just opaque in the center. With a wide spatula, transfer the fillets to a platter and sprinkle with **black sesame or chia seeds.**

MAKES 4 SERVINGS

Sautéed Monkfish Fillets

Total Time: 15 minutes

Cut **1 monkfish fillet (1½-pound),** dark membrane removed, into 4 pieces. Sprinkle the pieces with **sea salt** and **fresh or dried thyme or oregano** and **ground black pepper.** In a large skillet over medium-high heat, melt **1 tablespoon coconut oil.** Cook the fillets for 6 minutes, turning once, or until just opaque. Serve the fillets with **lime wedges.**

MAKES 4 SERVINGS

Shrimp Salad

Total Time: 10 minutes

In a large bowl, combine **1 package (8 ounces) frozen and thawed cooked baby shrimp, 1 small chopped apple, 1 small finely chopped red onion, 1 tablespoon olive oil or soy mayonnaise,** a **small handful chopped fresh dill or 1 tablespoon dried dill-weed,** and **ground black pepper.** Toss to coat well.

MAKES 4 SERVINGS

Variations:

- *Use canned tuna, crabmeat, lobster meat, or leftover chicken in place of the shrimp.*
- *Instead of the apple, incorporate a slice of sweet pineapple, canned peaches (drained and chopped), or a sliced pear.*
- *Add nuts or seeds like walnuts, sliced almonds, or sunflower seeds.*

Fruit

Fruit bought in season will be cheaper and better tasting; however, it's a little difficult these days to pinpoint exactly when a fruit's peak season is. Some fruits—such as strawberries—grow in all parts of the country and can truly be said to have a local growing season. But in most parts of the country, the vast majority of fruit in the market is imported from somewhere else. (There are no locally grown bananas in Michigan, for example.) In addition, much of the fruit grown in tropical and subtropical regions is available in our markets year-round. The "peak seasons" listed below merely represent times of the year when certain fruits are more abundant and, therefore, less expensive.

Fruit	Quantity for 4 Servings	Peak Season	Look for	Storage
Apples	4 medium	September–May	Firm flesh; unblemished skin; bright color for variety	Will keep 2 weeks.
Apricots	12 medium	June–July	Plump, juicy-looking fruit; smooth skin; bright golden orange color; flesh that yields to gentle pressure	Ripen at room temperature; will keep 3–5 days.
Avocados	2	Year-round	Pebbly, purple-black skin; flesh that feels slightly soft	Ripen at room temperature, refrigerate when ripe; will keep 3–5 days.
Bananas	4 medium	Year-round	Unblemished skin with or without brown speckles; yellow color	Ripen at room temperature; will keep 2–3 days.

	Fruit	Quantity for 4 Servings	Peak Season	Look for	Storage
Berries	Blackberries	1 pint	June–August	Plump berries; bright color for variety	Refrigerate, unwashed and uncovered; will keep 1–2 days.
	Blueberries	1 pint	May–August	Well-rounded shape; firm texture; dry skin; bright, purple-blue color with slightly frosted appearance	Refrigerate, unwashed and uncovered; will keep 5 days.
	Cranberries	1 pint	October–December	Firm texture; plump berries; high luster. (Good cranberries will bounce like rubber balls.)	Refrigerate, unwashed and uncovered; will keep 1–2 days.
	Raspberries	1 pint	June–August	Plump berries; bright color for variety	Refrigerate, unwashed and uncovered; will keep 1–2 days.
	Strawberries	4 cups (1 quart)	April–September	Firm texture; dry skin; vibrant red berries with bright green caps	Refrigerate, unwashed and uncovered; will keep 1–2 days.
Cherries, sour and sweet		1 pound	June–July	Firm fruit attached to stems; good color for variety	Refrigerate, unwashed and uncovered; will keep 1–2 days.

Fruit	Quantity for 4 Servings	Peak Season	Look for	Storage
Currants, fresh	1 pint	Midsummer	Firm texture; plump fruit; bright red, almost translucent color	Refrigerate, unwashed and uncovered; will keep 1–2 days.
Figs	4 medium	Midsummer	Slightly firm flesh; light yellow, reddish brown, or black color	Ripen in refrigerator; will keep 1–2 days.
Grapefruits	2 medium	Year-round	Fruits that seem heavy for their size; well-rounded shape; smooth, thin skin	Refrigerate; will keep 1–2 weeks.
Grapes	1–1½ pounds	Year-round	Plump fruit firmly attached to green, pliable stems; good color for variety	Refrigerate; will keep 4–6 days.
Guavas	1 pound	May–October	Depending on variety: pear or fig shape, red or yellow color	Ripen at room temperature, refrigerate when ripe; will keep 2–3 days.
Kiwifruit, green and golden	4 medium	Year-round (green), June–September (golden)	Firm fruit; fuzzy, brown skin	Ripen at room temperature, refrigerate when ripe; will keep 3–6 weeks.
Kumquats	10–12 medium	November–February	Fruits that seem heavy for their size; firm flesh; bright orange-yellow color	Refrigerate; will keep several days.

Fruit		Quantity for 4 Servings	Peak Season	Look for	Storage
Lemons		2 medium	Year-round	Fruits that seem heavy for their size; firm flesh; glossy, thin skin; light yellow color	Refrigerate; will keep 2 weeks.
Limes		2 medium	Year-round	Fruits that seem heavy for their size; firm flesh; glossy, thin skin; bright green color	Refrigerate; will keep 2 weeks.
Mangoes		2	May–August	Look for brightly colored skin and a sweet, fruity aroma. Flesh yields to gentle pressure.	Ripen at room temperature, refrigerate when ripe; will keep 2–3 days.
Melons	Muskmelons (cantaloupes, casaba, crenshaw, honeydew, Persian)	1–2 medium	May–October	Fruits that seem heavy for their size; pleasant, fruity aroma; color varies with variety; flesh that yields to slight pressure at blossom end	Ripen at room temperature, refrigerate, tightly wrapped, when ripe; will keep 2–3 days.
	Watermelon	¼ large	May–September	Smooth, velvety skin; creamy, not white or pale green, underside; firm, juicy flesh with good red or cream color; shiny, brown or black seeds	Refrigerate. Once cut, wrap exposed surface; will keep 1 week.

Fruit		Quantity for 4 Servings	Peak Season	Look for	Storage
Nectarines		4 medium	May–October	Firm flesh; plump fruit; smooth skin; reddish yellow color; slight softening along seam edge	Ripen at room temperature, refrigerate when ripe; will keep 3–5 days.
Oranges	Blood	4 medium	December–March	Fruits that seem heavy for their size; firm flesh; bright skin with a dark red blush	Refrigerate; will keep 2 weeks.
	Mandarin (clementine, tangelo, tangerine)	4 medium	November–March	Fruits that seem heavy for their size; firm flesh; loose skin. Tangerines: glossy skin.	Refrigerate; will keep 2 weeks.
	Sweet or juice	4 medium	Year-round	Fruits that seem heavy for their size; firm flesh; bright, smooth skin. Navel oranges are sweetest.	Refrigerate; will keep 2 weeks.
Papayas, organic only		1 large or 2 small	Year-round	Green (unripe) to bright orange or yellow (ripe) color; flesh that yields to gentle pressure	Ripen at room temperature, refrigerate when ripe; will keep 3–4 days.
Peaches		4 medium	May–October	Firm flesh that yields to gentle pressure; plump fruit; slightly fuzzy skin; white to yellow color with red blush	Ripen at room temperature, refrigerate when ripe; will keep 3–4 days.

Fruit	Quantity for 4 Servings	Peak Season	Look for	Storage
Pears	4 medium	Fall–winter	Firm flesh but starting to soften; plump fruit; color varies with variety	Ripen at room temperature, refrigerate when ripe; will keep 3–5 days.
Persimmons, Hachiya and Fuyu	4 medium	October–December	Hachiya: heart-shaped fruit; green stem caps; deep orange color. Fuyu: squat, tomato-shaped fruit; deep orange color.	Hachiya: Must be completely soft and ripe to be edible; ripen in a bag. Fuyu: Can be eaten when firm-ripe. Refrigerate when ripe; will keep 1–2 days.
Pineapples	1 large	Year-round	Large, heavy fruit; sweet aroma; depending on variety, green or golden yellow color; fresh, deep green crown leaves; nearly all eyes at base are yellow. Avoid pineapples with soft or discolored spots, watery or dark eyes, or brown leaves.	Refrigerate; will keep 1–2 days. If slightly under-ripe, keep at room temperature for several days.

Fruit	Quantity for 4 Servings	Peak Season	Look for	Storage
Plums	4 medium or 8 small	June–September	Plump fruit; good color for variety; flesh that yields to gentle pressure	Eat soon; will keep 3–5 days.
Pomegranates	4 medium	January–August	Fruits that seem heavy for their size; thin skin; purple-red color	Refrigerate; will keep 1 week.
Rhubarb	1 pound	February–May	Crisp, reddish green stalks	Refrigerate; will keep 3–5 days.

Fruit Recipes

Baked Apples

Total Time: 45 minutes

Preheat the oven to 350°F. Core **2 large apples** with a small knife, but do not cut all the way through to the bottoms. Peel about ½" of skin from the tops of the apples. Fill the apples evenly with **¼ cup melted ghee, 1 teaspoon cinnamon,** and a **few raisins.** Place them in a small baking dish. Cover the apples loosely with foil and bake for 30 minutes, or until the apples are tender.

MAKES 2 SERVINGS

Chocolate-Covered Banana

Total Time: 10 minutes + chilling time

Cut **1 peeled banana** in half lengthwise. Place each half on a small plate. In a small saucepan over low heat, heat **1 ounce dairy-free dark chocolate (70 percent cocoa or higher),** stirring frequently, for 3 minutes, or until the chocolate is melted and smooth. Evenly drizzle the melted chocolate over the banana halves. Refrigerate for 10 minutes, or until the chocolate is set.

MAKES 2 SERVINGS

Variations:

- *Use whole ripe organic strawberries or apple slices instead of a banana if you've already had some tropical fruit this week.*
- *You can also sauté half a banana in ghee, sprinkle it with cinnamon, and serve it hot for a different spin.*

Crustless Apple Pie

Total Time: 1 hour 30 minutes

Preheat the oven to 350°F. Core and thinly slice **4 large apples.** Place half of the slices in an 11" x 7" baking dish. Sprinkle the apples with a small **handful of chopped nuts and raisins.** Top with the remaining apple slices and another **small handful of chopped nuts and raisins.** Drizzle with **3 tablespoons melted ghee or coconut oil.** Cover loosely with foil and bake for 15 minutes, or until the apples are fragrant. Reduce the oven temperature to 300°F and bake for 1 hour, or until the apples are very tender. If you like, serve sprinkled with a **little dark rum** or with **Whipped Coconut Cream** (page 269).

MAKES 4 SERVINGS

Variations:

- *Use pears instead of apples for a different flavor.*
- *Try different types of nuts and seeds, like sunflower seeds, walnuts, sliced almonds, or hazelnuts.*
- *Instead of raisins, you can use dried cranberries, dried blueberries, or dried cherries.*

Fruit Smoothie   Total Time: 10 minutes

In a blender or food processor, combine **2 cored chopped apples, 1 frozen chopped banana or 1 chopped avocado, 1 cup sliced strawberries, 1 teaspoon chia seeds, 1 teaspoon grated fresh ginger,** and **1 cup coconut milk.** Blend until smooth.

MAKES 2 SERVINGS

Marinated Peaches   Total Time: 10 minutes + chilling time

In a medium bowl, combine **4 large peaches, pears, or apples (peeled, pitted or cored, and sliced), 1 pint fresh sliced straw- berries, 1 cup sparkling cider,** and **1 teaspoon ground cinna- mon.** Let stand in the refrigerator for 1 hour before serving.

MAKES 4 SERVINGS

Pineapple Mousse   Total Time: 10 minutes

Peel and cut ½ **ripe fresh pineapple** into chunks, place in a food pro- cessor (this recipe does not work in a blender), and process until foamy. If the pineapple is underripe, add a **few teaspoons maple syrup.** Serve immediately.

MAKES 4 SERVINGS

Poached Pears

Total Time: 20 minutes

In a large skillet, place **4 halved cored pears,** cut side up. Sprinkle with **1 to 2 tablespoons lemon juice.** Fill the pan with **1" of water** and add ½ **teaspoon vanilla extract** or ½ **teaspoon cinnamon.** Bring the water to a boil, and reduce the heat to low. Cover and simmer for 10 minutes, or until the pears are softened. Remove to a serving dish and drizzle with a bit of **melted ghee** (instead of sugar) and a **sprinkle of cinnamon.**

MAKES 4 SERVINGS

Vegetable Smoothie

Total Time: 10 minutes

In a blender or food processor, combine **2 to 3 cups frozen kale leaves, 1 rib celery, 1 chopped avocado,** ½ **cup goji berries or blueberries,** and **1 cup coconut milk or water.** Blend until thickened and smooth.

MAKES 2 SERVINGS

Variation:
- *Add fresh herbs and/or other fresh vegetables as desired.*

Sauces

Sometimes adding a little sauce can breathe new life into a familiar dish. If you find that you want to get a little creative, here are some favorite simple sauces to add some extra zest to your meals.

Chimichurri Sauce

Total Time: 5 minutes

In a food processor, combine ½ **cup parsley leaves, ¼ cup cilantro leaves, ¼ cup olive oil, 2 tablespoons red wine vinegar, 1 tablespoon lemon juice, ½ teaspoon dried oregano,** and **¼ teaspoon ground black pepper.** Process until blended. Store in an airtight container. Use 1 or 2 tablespoons as a condiment with lean meats and chicken.

MAKES 4 TO 6 SERVINGS

Green Sauce

Total Time: 10 minutes

In a food processor, combine **5 cloves garlic, 1 to 2 chopped carrots, 1 small chopped onion, ¼ to ½ cup fresh herbs (such as basil, dill, parsley, thyme, oregano, or cilantro), 1 to 4 teaspoons olive oil,** a **dash of sea salt** and a **dash of ground black pepper**. Process until smooth. Serve with fish, grains, or steamed vegetables. Freeze leftovers in an ice cube tray so it's always handy.

MAKES 8 TO 12 SERVINGS

Linden Flower Sauce

Total Time: 10 minutes + cooling time

Place a **handful of linden flowers** in a 2-cup glass measuring cup. Add **1 cup boiling water** and steep for 3 minutes. Strain the flowers out and let the water cool to room temperature. In a small bowl, whisk together **1 cup olive oil mayonnaise** and **1 to 2 tablespoons flower water** until it is the consistency of a sauce. Serve with fish.

MAKES 8–12 SERVINGS

Red Currant Sauce

Total Time: 5 minutes

In a small bowl, combine **¼ cup red currant jam, 2 teaspoons pre-pared mustard,** and a **pinch each of sea salt** and **ground black pepper.** This goes very well with all kinds of meats, including lamb, beef, and game meats.

MAKES 4 SERVINGS

Fresh Tomato Sauce

Total Time: 1 hour 15 minutes

In a large skillet over medium-high heat, melt **2 tablespoons coconut oil.** Cook **3 large chopped yellow onions** for 5 minutes, or until lightly browned. Add **6 to 8 minced cloves garlic, ¼ teaspoon sea salt,** and ¼ **teaspoon ground black pepper.** Add **6 to 8 pounds chopped fresh tomatoes, 1 can (5 ounces) sardines with bones, rinsed and drained,** and **1 tablespoon dried Italian seasoning.** Simmer for about 1 hour, or until the sauce thickens. Serve over **brown rice, beans,** or **quinoa.**

MAKES 8 TO 12 SERVINGS

Variations:

- *Use canned tuna in place of the sardines.*
- *Add 4 ounces ground beef for a different flavor.*
- *Add fresh herbs like oregano, marjoram, or mint.*

Whipped Coconut Cream

Total Time: 5 minutes + 1 hour chilling time

Open **1 can (14 ounces) organic unsweetened coconut milk (not lite)** and spoon the "full fat" coconut milk (the top half of can) into a chilled bowl. Transfer the remaining liquid in the can to a container and store in the refrigerator for later use. With an electric mixer on high speed, beat the coconut milk for 3 minutes, or until stiff peaks form. Cover and refrigerate for at least 1 hour, or until the coconut milk thickens.

MAKES 6 SERVINGS

Variations:

- *Serve cream on top of fresh ripe fruit like mangoes, peaches, apples, pears, oranges, blueberries, or cherries.*
- *Add cacao nibs for additional flavor.*

Natural Remedies for Common Diabetic Complaints

Keeping your body healthy is an expression of gratitude to the whole cosmos—the trees, the clouds, everything.

—THICH NHAT HANH (1926–)

If you have type 2 diabetes, you will experience diabetes-related complications, whether minor or major. And you'll also be more susceptible to developing other common ailments, so it is a good idea to know how to help yourself. Of course, you should not ditch your conventional physician. But ask if he or she is open to natural alternatives, and learn to apply methods from The Five Health Essentials. To get you started, I've compiled a list of the most common complaints from my patients, along with some natural remedies and suggestions for their relief and prevention. After all, achieving good health begins with prevention.

Aging

Aging and death are unavoidable. But for as long as you are living, you should have a good time and strive to leave the Earth a better place. All of the ideas in this book counteract premature aging, and there really is no difference in what keeps young or old people healthy: The methods I suggest aid both age groups.

Studies have shown that living a healthy, active life can actually postpone the aging process. So instead of buying a ton of "anti-aging" supplements or cosmetics that don't work, eat your greens, incorporate some movement into your life, get enough sleep, drink herbal teas and water, wash yourself down with a cold washcloth every evening, and stay involved with friends and family.[1-6] These are all great ways to keep premature aging at bay!

It's important to know that nearly everything in the plant world contributes to a longer, healthier life. But research has shown that certain anti-aging (and anti-diabetic) herbs and spices have the power of antioxidants to keep you energetic and perky for a bit longer.[7-8] Here are a few of my favorite herb and spice mixtures to delay the aging process.

- **Spice mixtures.** Curry is a blend of Indian spices, and its yellow color comes from the turmeric root. The most common ingredients in curry are turmeric, coriander (the seeds of cilantro), cumin, clove, fenugreek, and red pepper, but curries may also contain cinnamon, cardamom, caraway, black pepper, ginger, garlic, nutmeg, and more. There are hot and mild varieties, but all curries are antioxidant boosters. If you don't have an allergy to any of the ingredients, use this spice mixture frequently. Other mixtures with similar ingredients but surprisingly different tastes are apple pie spice, Chinese five-spice powder, pumpkin spice, Bengali Five-Spice, garam masala, chili powder, and cider mulling spices. So don't be afraid to experiment with any of these spices to see which tastes you prefer: They'll all help to keep you youthful and radiant.

- **Herbal mixtures.** Fines herbes (the classical mixture of French cuisine: tarragon, parsley, chervil, and chives), Italian seasoning, herbes de Provence, Greek herbs, Old Bay Seasoning (which contains herbs *and* spices), and Cajun herbs are all beneficial if you're looking to delay the aging process. Every ethnic kitchen and tradition has its own blend of herbal mixtures, and you can recreate these flavors in your kitchen. *Note:* Don't buy herb and spice mixtures that contain salt, MSG, or unnatural additions. Go for the real thing.

- **Herbal tea mixtures.** Teas and tisanes (herbal teas with no caffeine) keep your cells hydrated and young. The possibilities to combine caffeinated and noncaffeinated teas with herbs are endless: Masala chai (and many other chai mixtures), Earl Grey, rooibos with bergamot (a noncaffeinated version of Earl Grey), Moroccan tea (any mixture with mint in it), Rote Grütze (a berry mix from Germany), and coconut chai are some excellent options. And don't forget that you can purchase ready-made mixtures that fight all kinds of minor ailments, such as coughs and colds, urinary tract infections, hay fever, sleeplessness, female troubles, and more.

Alzheimer's Disease and Dementia

While there is a genetic link in the development of Alzheimer's disease, certain habits can either promote or fight dementia. Eating sugar and bad fats and skipping vegetables bodes poorly for your mental health in older age. But research has shown that doing moderate exercise brings blood to your brain, which delays intellectual decline.[9] And like taking a cold shower or eating anti-inflammatory foods, the effects of exercise last only as long as you keep up the habit. Once you stop, they wear off quickly.

In terms of dietary support, it comes down to this: What is good against diabetes is good against Alzheimer's, heart disease, cancer, and more. Returning to the dietary needs and activities our bodies were designed for keeps us healthy and sharp into old age. But there is even more to the relationship between diabetes and Alzheimer's: Your brain—to scientists' surprise—produces a bit of insulin. This insulin in your brain not only serves to lower sugar, it also regulates and transfers signals in your brain,[10] and interrupted signal transfer can lead to dementia. High blood sugar interferes with the small amount of insulin production in your brain, muffling the brain signals and the signals from cell to cell. Your brain reacts to this in phases, similar to those that your pancreas goes through: First there is an overproduction, with insulin resistance and leptin resistance. Then comes underproduction and, in the case of your brain, dementia.

So what does this all mean? By following the plan provided in this book, you'll not only reverse or even cure your diabetes, but you'll also help your body to stave off dementia.

Arterial Disease

High blood sugar damages arterial vessel walls, which causes narrowing of your arteries. This is one of the dreaded complications of advanced diabetes, as toe, foot, or leg infections often require amputation. You can prevent arterial disease if you tackle your diabetes early on. But if you let your diabetes linger, the outcome might be dismal. To prevent arterial disease, get your diabetes under control by eating an anti-inflammatory diet, walking and taking the stairs as often as you can, and including daily anti-inflammatory supplements like fish oil and zinc.

Arthritis (Osteoarthritis)

Most people think arthritis is a normal part of aging, but that's not true. Arthritis is linked to our Western nutrition patterns and can be prevented, and even ameliorated, later in life. To improve or prevent arthritis, avoid sugar, gluten, and dairy. (The proteins in dairy only worsen the inflammation in your joints.) Focus on staying active throughout the day, and avoid sitting for prolonged periods of time. Make sure to eat plenty of vegetables— except nightshades (tomatoes, potatoes, eggplant, and hot and bell peppers). And if you need additional support, taking the supplement glucosamine helps in 40 percent of cases, but you have to take it for at least 6 months before you see any results. Research has also shown that the omega-3 fatty acids in fish oil can help to improve your condition.[11]

Athlete's Foot

Fungus likes dark, warm, moist, and sweet places—and that is why undercover, in America's shoes, nail fungus is attacking like body snatchers. To call it "athlete's foot" is giving nail fungus a misleadingly nice name. Think about it in terms of germs invading a body after death: Nail fungus is invading your body *before* death!

It's a common belief that we get the fungus because we catch it from public spaces like pools and hotel rooms. But the truth is, the offending fungus spores—most often those of *Trichophyton rubrum*—are everywhere and are impossible to avoid. Still, nail fungus was uncommon only a few generations ago. Today, we pick up the offenders because our bodies' defenses are lowered by a diet high in sugar.

So if nail fungus grows in dark, warm, moist, and sweet places, let's spoil it for the invaders and make the location bright, cool, dry, and decidedly unsweet! Wear light, airy shoes whenever possible. If you have to wear heavy boots or sneakers, use ample baby powder for dryness, and change your shoes and socks often. You can microwave your shoes after wearing them, but only if there are no metal buckles on them. Begin with less than a minute, because some modern materials melt and blister, and work up to as long as 1 minute. Alternatively, dust your shoes with foot powder right after slipping out of them. Also, walk around barefoot at home to air out your feet, or wear slip-resistant socks, but no shoes.

There are many natural methods to fight nail fungus, usually involving essential oils and/or garlic. The following method is highly effective (unless you are allergic to any of the ingredients): Rub your feet and nails twice a day with coconut oil and tea tree oil. Or apply olive oil with a drop of thyme, oregano, or rosemary oil. Repeat this twice a day until all signs of fungus are gone, then continue once daily to prevent a recurrence. Keep in mind that whenever you eat something sweet, your nail fungus thrives. So don't feed the invader. Instead, build a shield around you by eating a diet high in vegetables.

Back Pain

There are many causes of back pain, and to resolve most of them, you need a doctor and good imaging of your skeleton. But sometimes the cure is simple, as in the examples below.

Example 1: When I was young and living in Germany, I complained to a doctor about upper back pain. He slid his gaze from my head to my toes and curtly said, "No wonder—with those flat feet." As a result of this visit, I got orthotic inserts, and the problem was gone.

Example 2: A neighbor came to visit and complained of acute back pain, so I sent him to a Trager practitioner. (Trager is a form of gentle bodywork that aligns your spine and your joints.)[12]

The neighbor returned later with his son to tell me about the miraculous treatment. The practitioner seemed to think this was not a herniated disc, but a sacrum problem. While talking with the father, I offered his son a piece of dark milk-free chocolate; the boy declined politely because he'd just had chocolate—with nuts. The father bragged that he was eating a lot of nuts now, for health—especially cashews. This sent up a red flag because cashews are in the same family as poison ivy (Anacardiaceae, or the sumac family). It is well known for inducing inflammation in the body—especially in the back and joints. So I immediately knew the diagnosis: cashew-induced sacroiliitis.

Besides Trager movement education, I recommended Zyflamend (an expensive—but well worth it—herbal concoction available at your local health food store). Zyflamend has great anti-inflammatory action—if you aren't allergic to any of the dozen herbal ingredients. And, needless to say, no more cashews (or mangoes, which also belong to the same family). The neighbor was cured in 2 days.

So if you find yourself suffering from back pain, try a few of the suggestions listed above. But if these don't help you find relief soon, pay a visit to your physician to uncover the root cause of your pain.

Blindness

Diabetes often leads to visual impairment and, ultimately, blindness. The most frequent cause is diabetic retinopathy, where the small vessels in your eye are affected (not surprisingly; we've discussed how diabetes hurts your vessel walls). In one small study, researchers divided patients into three different groups: prediabetics, early diabetics, and full-blown diabetics. They then tested all of the groups with *laser scanning Doppler flowmetry*. The scary conclusion was that the three groups all showed the same amount of damage to their retinas.[13] This confirms the idea that conventional medicine diagnoses diabetes too late and that injury is already occurring before we even suspect it. But diabetics have other eye afflictions, too—and all of them in higher numbers than nondiabetics: vitreous detachment, retinal detachment, macular degeneration, cataract, and glaucoma.[14–18]

A Chinese study looked at the diabetics who were most likely to lose their eyesight during the course of their diabetes. Those patients were more likely to be older and had diabetes longer, had higher A1c results, and had higher blood pressure. But the test in which they differed most was microalbuminuria—a urine dipstick test that shows whether or not your kidneys are in danger.[19] People with a positive dipstick test were twice as likely to develop the dreaded diabetic retinopathy. So, unfortunately, the patients who might end up on dialysis are also the ones who will go blind.

Here's what you can do: Eat as many vegetables as possible and avoid sugar, dairy, and trans fats. Add good fats to your dishes and make sure your bowels and liver are healthy, resulting in good digestion. Always wear eye protection when you're out in the sun. In addition, taking a supplement that's high in antioxidants (like Gaia Herbs Vision Enhancement phyto-caps, or any reputable brand of vision antioxidants) might help prevent or delay macular degeneration.

Boils

A boil is a pimple, only bigger and more painful, and in diabetics they occur after the teenage years are over. The medical terms are *furuncle* or *carbuncle*— deep infections of the hair follicle (the little sac out of which the hair grows); carbuncles are bigger, with several heads. Both usually harbor staphylococcus bacteria.

Boils are one sign that your blood sugar may be too high. When a nondiabetic gets frequent boils, it is a sign that his or her immune system isn't functioning well. In the early stages, you can try to make a boil go away by applying tea tree oil and/or coconut oil after each shower or bath, or as needed, up to two or three times a day. Both oils have antibacterial properties and soak in quickly—just wipe off any excess.

Once a boil comes to a head, though, it is better to see a doctor, because it may need to be cut and drained. Neglected boils can fester and spread the infection to other parts of your body, like your brain and bones, or they can lead to deadly sepsis.

Cancer

Research has shown that cancer occurs more often in those who are obese and have type 2 diabetes.[20-21] It's not because diabetics produce more cancer cells—we all constantly develop microscopic cancer cells, but a healthy immune system will typically gobble them up. But a diabetic's body will feed those cancer cells better than a healthy body: A sugary environment is heaven for cancer cells.

In prehistoric times, and even in most historic times, cancer was a rare event—and not because people died at a younger age. The ones who survived starvation, accidents, and homicide actually lived to the same ripe old ages that we do now. Today, roughly a quarter of Americans die of cancer, and medicine and research have barely put a dent in the statistics. This isn't because modern science hasn't advanced, but because our lifestyle deviates more than ever from what Nature intended for us. We are now exposed to chemicals alien to our ancient bodies, chemicals that interrupt all kinds of natural processes, from reproduction to the repair of DNA. Instead of roaming around, we are sitting all day. And without daily access to natural light to sustain us, our cancer cells thrive.

Interestingly, metformin, one of the main diabetes drugs, seems to help cancer patients to survive longer.[22] And there is one cancer that is less common in patients with type 2 diabetes: prostate cancer, thanks to lower testosterone levels in diabetics.[23] To me, the price seems a bit high to pay for *that* advantage.

It has been speculated that insulin resistance plays a role in cancer development more than insulin per se. On the other hand, insulin has a powerful molecular cousin called *insulin-like growth factor 1*, which is stimulated by growth hormones and might foster cancer cell growth. And wouldn't you know it? Growth hormones are now added systematically to milk and other dairy products.

So what have you done *today* to ward off those tiny enemy cells? Research has shown that exercise protects against cancer. So go rake some leaves in the yard or go for a walk. And remember that light also protects you from cancer via vitamin D, which is created under your skin when you are exposed to sunlight. Just make sure to prevent sunburns to avoid the risk of skin cancer.

In terms of diet, starve your cancer by depriving it of sugar! Studies have found that without sugar, cancer cells will die.[24] It might also help to eat some cod liver once a month, as this gives you a good dose of vitamin D. As an alternative, get a good old-fashioned cod liver oil supplement or some vitamin D capsules: 1,000 milligrams is a moderate daily dose if your levels are on the lower side.

You should also eat as many vegetables as you can get your hands on. Broccoli is in the cruciferous family (another name for the cabbage family). Most cabbages contain cancer-fighting compounds. Horseradish belongs in this group, as well as Brussels sprouts, savoy cabbage, bok choy, and so many more.

If you already have cancer, shock your system—and the cancer cells—with as many vegetables, herbs, and phytonutrients as you can eat. You might prolong your life that way, because everything that is good for diabetics is perfect nutrition for cancer patients.

Candidiasis of the Mouth

Also called a yeast infection or thrush, it often occurs in people with reduced immune capability and those who've just been treated with antibiotics. It presents as little white spots or redness in the mouth, or deeper down in the esophagus as pain when swallowing and eating. If your doctor has confirmed the diagnosis, you can try this at home: Mix ½ teaspoon salt and ½ teaspoon turmeric in a glass of warm water. Swish it around in your mouth and gargle for a few seconds before spitting it out. Repeat several times a day. This also relieves a sore throat. (*Note:* When taken alone—without the salt—tumeric may help to relieve esophageal thrush and can be swallowed.)

Cellulite

Cellulite (in medical terminology: gynoid lipodystrophy) is a dreaded nuisance for many women, presenting as dimpled masses of fat around the thighs. Although a study showed that people who were severely overweight improved their cellulite when they lost weight, those who weighed less at the beginning of the experiment experienced worse cellulite after weight loss. So what is a woman to do?

The Natural Medicine take on cellulite is that it is poorly exercised, inflamed fat. But the good news is: There's hope! Here's what you can do to combat those unsightly dimples.

- Eliminate all dairy products (cheese, butter, yogurt, and milk) from your diet. Dairy seems to be the one single aggravating factor for cellulite.

- Focus on eating an anti-inflammatory diet, as outlined in Chapter 7.

- If you don't already exercise, start with a very moderate exercise program (intense programs don't work; they will only overwhelm you). Check out the easy 1-minute movements from Chapter 9. You can even invent some new exercises yourself—just move!

- Brush your skin with a dry brush, always in the direction of your heart. It is not as effective as exercise, but it mobilizes those sluggish fat cells. And don't even think about buying those anticellulite creams—they don't work and are a waste of money!

- Always end your hot shower with a short cold one.

Andrographis Paniculata: The Wonder Herb

When fighting a cold, or any ailment that causes a tickling sensation in your throat or nose, look no further than your local herbal or health store. There, on the shelf, you'll find an amazing herbal supplement called *Andrographis paniculata.* So what makes this herb so great? It basically makes the mucosa of your upper airways uninhabitable for viruses. And by reducing mucus, it also helps tremendously in treating asthma, hay fever, and sinusitis.

I found *Andrographis paniculata* while traveling in Australia: Within a few hours of arriving in Melbourne, I came down with what promised to be an exceptionally nasty cold—probably something I picked up on the airplane. We only had a few days for sightseeing and visiting friends, and I was desperate not to be sick in a hotel bed. At the local drugstore, I asked for an herbal medication that would fight my oncoming cold. The pharmacist explained that their establishment did not carry something as unscientific as herbs and offered a row of the usual over-the-counter cough medications, which I did not want to take. When I insisted that, surely, there had to be some herbs in his store, he produced a colorful little box and said, "My Chinese customers buy these." I bought them, took a few of those tiny pills called Chuan Xin Lian Pian, and 2 hours later I was on my way to recovery. It worked like a charm!

Later I learned that this formula contained the wonder herb *Andrographis paniculata.* Since then, this inexpensive supplement has become my standard cold medication. In Ayurvedic medicine, *Andrographis paniculata* is called Maha-tita ("King of bitters") because of its bitter taste (which you will barely notice if you take it as a capsule). It is just another example of the health benefits of bitters. Aiding digestion along is one of *Andrographis paniculata's* primary uses. It is also strongly anti-inflammatory and has antiviral, antibacterial, and antifungal properties. In Chinese medicine it is prescribed for lung support in cold conditions—just what I needed that day in Melbourne.

Cellulite is not a beauty problem. It is a quick measure of your metabolic health. While a little bit of dimpling might just come with age, the symptom that annoys you now might, in the long run, present as heart disease, diabetes, stroke, dementia, arthritis, depression, and cancer.

Colds

There may not be a cure for the common cold, but there are a few things you can do to shorten the amount of time you'll spend suffering from the symptoms. See the list below for a few tips.

- At the first sign of a cold, go to bed early. Sleep is paramount for a working immune system.
- Drink a lot of hot fluids. Liquids like unsweetened elderberry juice, herbal teas, and lemon juice with organic unheated honey are particularly soothing.
- Avoid eating sugary foods, as sugar only feeds the bugs. If you have no appetite, don't force yourself to eat.
- Rinse your nose with saltwater (see Chapter 11).
- Take *Andrographis paniculata*. This herbal supplement is my favorite remedy to nip a cold in the bud, as it has few negative side effects— and many positive effects. Take two capsules every 3 to 4 hours until your symptoms are gone. For more information, see "*Andrographis Paniculata*: The Wonder Herb" (opposite).

Constipation/Diarrhea

What constitutes a healthy bowel? A healthy bowel movement: Your bowels should move at least once a day. If you don't have a bowel movement every day, don't reach for a laxative. Instead, take a look at your diet. Do you eat enough vegetables and fruits? What about beans and lentils, for fiber? Leave out sugar, trans fats, and dairy. And don't eat anything that causes stomach pain, heartburn, bloating, cramps, or sores in your mouth—these are all signs that something is hurting your digestion. You may also take a probiotic, which will help restore healthy bowel flora, but don't assume that this makes up for eating a lousy diet. Taking a probiotic should only supplement your new, healthy, anti-inflammatory diet.

Dupuytren's Contracture

Dupuytren's contracture is a hardening of the fascia in the palm of the hand that leads to a contracture of the fingers—most often the fourth (or ring) finger. If you have this condition, you can see and feel the hard string right under your skin. Often, the nondominant hand is involved, but I have seen it in both hands in my patients.

The cause of Dupuytren is unknown, but it clearly runs in families and seems to be linked to diabetes, abnormal blood fats, dairy consumption, and increased alcohol consumption. It occurs more often in people of Scandinavian descent and is 10 times more common in men than in women. (A similar affliction of the penis is called Peyronie's disease. One side of the penis shaft gets hardened, which leads to a permanent bend in the organ. What helps treat Dupuytren will also help with Peyronie's.)

Dupuytren is one of those diseases that seem to affect only a small part of your body—that funny area there in your hand—but, in reality, it's a systemic disease, affecting many more organs. I view Dupuytren as a metabolic disorder, so getting your lipids under control is of utmost importance. A diet high in vegetables and herbs and containing no fried foods or dairy, small amounts of meat, and no alcohol can soften the hardened fascia and reverse the process.

Earwax

You know that you shouldn't clean your ears with cotton swabs, and I have told this to my patients a thousand times. Why, then, do I find myself turning the little white swab in my ear canal after each shower? I don't advise doing this because it can cause damage to your eardrum. But if you insist on doing it, don't push it too far into your ear and use a dab of virgin coconut oil on the end of the swab. It is bactericidal and fungicidal, and your ears will stop itching immediately. And what about ear candling, which has become popular in the last few years? There is not a single scientific study proving its efficacy, or even its mechanisms. There have, however, been a few bad outcomes from burns.[25]

Flu

If you've been diagnosed with diabetes, you need to take extra precautions during flu season. Below are the three most common questions I've received about flu season and how to protect yourself during that time.

Do I need to get a flu shot?

If anyone needs a flu shot, diabetics do. Of course, I want you to focus on healing your body naturally, but if your A1c is above 6.0, you should definitely get this shot. Also heart patients, asthmatics, and those who have a chronic disease or struggle with obesity are more susceptible to the complications of the flu, so the flu shot is necessary for them, as well. There are two problems, though. First, according to the *Center for Disease Control and Prevention*, the vaccine is not as effective in the elderly due to their weaker immune systems,and it happens that being older and being diabetic often run together.[26] Second, multiple-dose flu shots contain preservatives, most often thimerosal, which is a mercury compound. In the best situation, we would all get single-dose flu shots that don't require thimerosal, but these are expensive. If you have asthma, hay fever, eczema, or allergies, you should talk your doctor about the single-dose vaccine.

How do I keep from getting the flu?

Thinking they have now done what they could by getting a flu shot, many people never take the responsibility for their health into their own hands. Much illness—and even many infections—can be prevented by nurturing a vigorous body and maintaining good health habits. The most important thing you can do during flu season is get enough sleep: 8 to 9 hours on average (not more). If your system is run-down, you will catch what flies around in the air. The good news is that if you follow The Five Health Essentials, you have everything you need to fight flu season because you're already building up your immune system.

Before flu season begins, ask your physician to check your vitamin D level to determine whether you're getting enough of the valuable vitamin. During the winter, we deplete our stores of vitamin D and eat fewer foods rich in vitamin D, which leads to increased susceptibility to infections. Why? We tend to stay indoors more and we eat more—and decreased movement and unhealthy holiday foods weaken your body.

Are there any herbal treatments I can use to stave off the flu?

Every few hours during a bad outbreak, chew on fresh garlic cloves. Take a lick of unheated honey (Manuka is the best) every hour or so; it kills germs. (But don't use it for children under 3 years old—there's a risk of botulism!) Take the following as supplements: a probiotic, fish oil, and vitamin D. Also, rinse your nose with saltwater (see page 176) prophylactically and when it is stuffed, to kill germs. (Carefully rinse your mouth afterward with clear water if you have high blood pressure.)

Foot Care

Diabetics often have poor circulation, which means that a minor wound can easily turn into a major infection. But with peripheral neuropathy and decreased pain perception, a diabetic may not realize that something is wrong. This is why daily inspection of your feet is so important. But when your eyesight is failing, you can't do this well—and a combination of these conditions conspires to lead to amputations.

If your eyesight is poor, don't cut your own toenails—get a pedicure. Use tea tree oil, aloe gel, or neem oil on minor wounds. Rub your feet every day with virgin coconut oil to keep the skin healthy and to fight germs. On festering diabetic wounds and ulcers, I would use honey to kill the germs—especially Manuka honey. Use caution with aloe if the wound is more than superficial. (Deep wounds can be closed too early by aloe vera's great healing power.) And make sure you visit an emergency room or your physician immediately if something feels wrong: Never delay, because the consequences can be dire.

Heatstroke

During the worst of the hot, hot summer nights, my husband and I have a simple fan running in the bedroom. Why, you may ask? When summer is

The Power of Neem Oil

Neem oil comes from the fruit and seeds of the Indian tree *Azadirachta indica,* and one of its Indian names is "village pharmacy," as it seems to heal just about everything. In India, its young, bitter leaves are eaten as a vegetable, but I wouldn't recommend neem oil internally because it has also been approved as a pesticide. And if it works to kill garden germs, it is only logical that it might also kill your body's cells. Neem oil has also been linked to liver toxicity, especially in children. And in men, eating neem leaves leads to temporary infertility, which is reversed when one stops eating the leaves. So do not use neem internally unless you are working with an herbalist or physician.

That said, neem oil is one of the best herbal antimicrobials and is, therefore, useful against the small wounds that so often seem incurable in diabetics and can easily lead to major catastrophes. In fact, a recent study showed that using a combination of St. John's wort extract with neem oil was effective in treating diabetic foot wounds.[16] Make sure to always have neem oil on hand, as I do, to treat minor cuts and abrasions. So head out to your local health food or herbal store and pick up a bottle of this helpful solution.

upon us, we savor every minute of it by slowing down, relaxing, and taking it easy. And sweating. Sweating is the natural, seasonal way to detoxify. I'm not saying you should never enjoy the comfort of air conditioners: I think at the workplace, they help people concentrate on their work instead of idly looking out of the window. And I don't want to discuss the possible health disadvantages of air conditioning here—I just want to encourage you to give your body a chance to naturally detoxify, which will help to build up your immune system.

I am aware that some areas are much hotter than where I live. If this is true for your location, it's important to avoid heatstroke. Stay in the shade, keep activity to a minimum, drink plenty of lukewarm fluids (like lightly steeped black tea with mint), splash your face and arms with cold water, and if you don't have an air conditioner, hang up moist towels: The evaporation will cool your surroundings.

Irritable Bowel Syndrome (IBS)

In my 30 years as a physician, I have never diagnosed anybody with "irritable bowel syndrome," or IBS. It's not that I didn't want to make the diagnosis, but it always seemed to be the last resort, only made if there wasn't a better explanation for the patient's symptoms. And there always was.

If my patients came with that label, I quietly looked for a more appropriate diagnosis, mostly some kind of food intolerance and/or infection. I believed that if they came to me with any of the myriad of gastrointestinal complaints that fall under the umbrella of IBS, they deserved a thorough workup. Physicians discern between food allergies and food intolerances. But for the patient, the difference is minimal: The only action that will help is removing the offending food from your diet. Allergies are mediated either through blood (they show up in blood tests) or through cells (meaning they can't be detected by blood tests). If the latter is determined, a skin prick test is the way to go. But in most cases, the tests are largely unnecessary because your body will signal what is wrong.

If you usually feel good (or even just better) in the morning before you eat, it's likely you have a food allergy or intolerance. Floating or large stools, bloating, and excessive gas also point to a food culprit, too. You should always see a physician if you suspect that your IBS is a result of a food intolerance, but there are some helpful things you can do to get some relief in the meantime.

- Keep a food journal. Everything that goes into your mouth should be listed, including beverages, pills, and chewing gum. A pattern might become clear once you record everything regularly.

- Read labels! Of course, foods without labels—like kale and carrots—are healthier anyway because only processed food is required to be labeled.

- Jot down any pain or issues like headaches, heartburn, stomachaches, bloating, diarrhea, constipation, blurred vision, slow urination, skin rashes, sneezing, wheezing, dark circles under your eyes, and stuffy nose or ears that occur after eating.

- Don't eat after dinner, and don't have dinner late—give your stomach a rest. The sheer bulk in your stomach may create discomfort. Besides, eating late prevents cell repair that should be taking place nightly but that can't happen when your body is busy digesting.

- If you suspect food allergies, remove the most common offenders (dairy, soy, nuts, gluten, corn, nightshades, citrus fruit, seafood, lectins, food colorings, preservatives, flavor enhancers and colors, eggs, apples and other fruits, chocolate, and yeast) plus whatever you suspect for a week. Then, every week, reintroduce one food from the list. Sometimes only repeated exposure shows the problem—and that happens mostly with cell-mediated allergies.
- Never try to force your body into accepting any food that it doesn't want! Blood-mediated allergies are fast-acting and can require a trip to the emergency room (peanut allergies are one example).
- Take a probiotic preparation regularly. As there are different beneficial gut bacteria, change brands and strains frequently. Begin with a small dose and slowly increase your dosage. If a probiotic does not agree with you, change brands.
- Most people benefit from fish oil, which counteracts the constant inflammation that comes with food allergies.
- Chew your food well.
- Eat vegetables, vegetables, and more vegetables. Not only are they good for you, but they also seem to cause fewer allergies.
- Stop running for a while, if that's your exercise of choice. About 50 percent of serious runners suffer from a curious disease called runner's diarrhea, so give yourself a break and see if your problem clears up on its own.

Unfortunately, you can have a bowel disease without any gastrointestinal complaints: About 50 percent of gluten intolerance (celiac sprue) patients never notice anything wrong with their bellies. But they might have joint or back pain, diabetes, neuropathy, autoimmune disease, mental fog, depression, schizophrenia, and a host of other problems. So stay aware of your body and any changes that may occur—and report them to your doctor.

Osteoporosis

Bones contain calcium, potassium, manganese, magnesium, silica, iron, zinc, selenium, boron, phosphorus, sulfur, chromium, and more—but the dairy industry tries to tell us that all we need for strong bones is calcium. Doesn't sound accurate, does it?

We've already discussed how vegetables contain enough calcium for strong bones. Plus they contain all the other minerals our bodies require for healthy bones. We don't need fortified, adulterated, hormone-injected dairy products for our bones. Also, our official daily requirements for calcium seem to be set artificially high: In one study in Africa, women took in only about half the recommended dose and maintained excellent bone health.[28]

Another problem with dairy is that it provides protein, and the standard American diet (SAD) contains too much protein as it is. We are omnivores by nature; once in a while a piece of meat between our teeth provides us with essential nutrients that are hard to come by otherwise, like vitamin B_{12}. But one existing hypothesis is that consuming too much protein leaches calcium from our bones because the metabolic products of protein digestion are acidic and need alkaline compounds for buffering. Regardless of whether or not this hypothesis is true, diets high in protein (meats and dairy) have been linked to osteoporosis.

Lists comparing the calcium content of dairy with vegetables often show higher values for dairy products. What these lists don't tell you is that calcium from plants (fruit, vegetables, grains, legumes, nuts—everything that has grown) absorbs at the same rate as the calcium from dairy[29-30]—without the extra calories and extra protein burden.

So what about calcium supplements? Don't think you'll get much benefit from them: Number one, the calcium without the other minerals will not do you much good. Number two, as a physician, I am all too familiar with that oblong white spot on an x-ray of the bowels: the unabsorbed calcium pill. You're better off putting your money into fresh produce. So if you really want to fight osteoporosis, eat your greens and go for daily walks, as research has shown that both moderate exercise and exposure to sunlight aid in building strong bones.

Pain

Another medical shortcut I stopped believing in long ago: If you're in pain, just pop a painkiller. If a simple pain reliever will do the trick, the pain is probably not intolerable. Serious pain—it goes without saying—needs the attention of a physician. But for minor aches and pains—especially joint pains—you can use willow bark, cat's claw, and glucosamine supplements, which have fewer side effects. (Find these at your local health food store and follow the dosage directions on the bottles.) Migraines can be prevented, in many cases, by regularly taking feverfew supplements, while other headaches may be prevented by increasing the amount of exercise you get, participating in Trager bodywork, maintaining better posture, and getting sufficient sleep.

Parkinson's Disease

Parkinson's is too complicated an issue to discuss at length here. There certainly is a genetic component, but lifestyle choices can trigger Parkinson's prematurely. What I have found with my patients is that what helps with diabetes also helps with Parkinson's—especially removing dairy (and often gluten) from your diet, moving moderately, eating an anti-inflammatory diet, and avoiding trans fats and artificial molecules, especially sweeteners.

Reflux

This is one of those ailments that keep people on medication forever—and on the face of it, there's no cure. In the long run, it can be a dangerous disease because long-standing erosion of the esophagus can lead to Barrett's esophagus and even cancer. But why are so many people living with the diagnosis of reflux?

Reflux is, in most instances, another disease resulting from the standard American diet (SAD). People have intolerances to certain foods and allergies, and those keep the esophagus (and possibly the stomach and the whole gut) inflamed. Instead of having the patient eliminate the offending foods, the doctor prescribes Zantac or Tagamet, or even one of the stronger proton pump inhibitors (PPIs). And by doing this, that doctor has gained a lifelong patient.

Unfortunately, those stomach medications create new problems: Because they all reduce acidity, they may also hinder digestion and further infections, as stomach acid is supposed to kill invading germs. PPIs (drugs like Prilosec, Prevacid, and Nexium), the strongest antiheartburn medications, can also be addictive, trigger food allergies, and weaken your bones. Recently the FDA also sent out warnings about pneumonia in connection with PPIs.

Heartburn is rarely caused by too much acidity for no good reason. (That condition is called Zollinger-Ellison syndrome, and it should be ruled out by your doctor if the burning goes on relentlessly, regardless of what you do.)

Normally, your stomach reacts with pain when you eat something wrong or overindulge in certain foods. So why not get to the underlying cause? Sometimes physicians diagnose a hiatal hernia in conjunction with reflux—a gap in your diaphragm that allows the stomach to move up a bit into your chest area. But no connection has been found between this and reflux. It seems that many people have a hiatal hernia, either for unknown reasons or because they're carrying a paunch that pushes their organs up into their chest cavity.

If you're tired of experiencing reflux on a regular basis, find out which foods your body cannot tolerate. It's not difficult; all you have to do is keep track of your meals in a food journal to notice what dishes are making you sick. Things to note include:

- **Any pharmaceutical drugs you are taking.** Most medications come with side effects. Could your reflux be one of them? Note when you take your medication and when your reflux occurs.

- **How your food is prepared.** Is it raw or cooked? Usually, cooked is easier on the stomach, and you get more nutrients out of your fare. So make a note of any raw foods you're eating. You may be able to keep a favorite food but just change the way you prepare it.

- **The timing of your reflux.** Some people get away with a raw salad or an acidic fruit during the day, but not at night, as the last meal that lingers in their stomach.

- **Patterns of reflux after consuming certain food groups.** You could be allergic to a whole food group! Many people do better without nightshades, sugars, and white starches and with a reduced intake of whole grains.

- **All junk foods and processed foods.** All of these should be under suspicion. They contain trans fats and preservatives, as well as colorings, stabilizers, and flavorings that are alien to your body.

- **Your water intake.** Are you getting enough fluid, and what does your hydration schedule look like? Drink plenty of water (see Chapter 11), but not with meals or right afterward.

If you're looking for more immediate relief from reflux, take a look at these healing herbs and supplements.

- Mastic gum is an agent that coats your stomach and helps if you have been indiscreet, food-wise. Unfortunately, mastic is not cheap. An alternative, which may be paid for by insurance, is Carafate, which has a similar action. Take it away from meals.

- Deglycyrrhizinated licorice (DGL) helps. Because it is deglycyrrhized, it does not have the effect of increasing your blood pressure. It also comes as a lozenge.

- Other herbs that soothe your stomach are chamomile tea and the jellylike inside of the aloe vera leaf, eaten directly from the plant (but avoid the green outside leaf—it is a harsh laxative), slippery elm, plantain banana, calendula, marshmallow (the herb—not the sweet candy!), cabbage juice, and artichoke extract. But be aware of your own body: I, for instance, have a chamomile allergy, so it would not soothe *my* stomach!

In addition to tracking your dietary patterns and taking supplements or herbs, avoid the following:

- Big, heavy meals
- Eating after dinner
- Peppermint, as it has a relaxing effect on the sphincter that closes the stomach

Sinus Problems

Most sinus infections are caused by allergies, bacteria, and fungi. And since germs are fed by a sweet diet, diabetics, with their elevated blood sugars, are naturally more prone to those problems than the rest of the population. Here are a few tips for treating chronic sinusitis.

- Avoid all milk and dairy products, as they are mucus producing.
- Avoid ice-cold beverages because they can trigger sneezing attacks and exacerbate asthma. Instead, drink hot beverages with lemon and honey, which seem to soothe chronic sinusitis. Herbal teas are helpful in healing the sinuses, as well.
- Interestingly, getting chilly might affect some people with chronic conditions. Avoid cold drafts and try to stay in warmer environments.
- Exhaustion depletes immune function, so focus on getting enough rest and sleep. This is especially important for children and adolescents.

- Avoid spicy foods, which will only aggravate the condition, and look for possible food allergies that could trigger sinus activity.

Skin, Dry and Itchy

If you're prone to dry and itchy skin and your regular lotion doesn't do the trick, perhaps it's time to look elsewhere—such as in your kitchen! Coconut oil is one of the most soothing options you can use on your skin, and it can be incredibly helpful in providing relief from itchy, dry skin. Use it in place of your standard body lotion after each shower or bath to restore moisture to your skin, or any other time your skin feels dry. It soaks in quickly, and don't worry about applying too much: Just wipe off any excess that isn't absorbed.

Tooth Health

Two common tooth problems are cavities (tooth decay) and parodontosis (gum disease). When gum disease worsens, it loosens your teeth (and is then called periodontitis); one can lose a perfectly healthy tooth just because it lost its grip on the bone (or the other way around).

Herbs. For a while I went to regular dental appointments. But the brutality with which they used sharp instruments to remove plaque appalled me; there is nothing natural about that process, as "primitive" people had healthy teeth because of their sugar-free diets. I got myself a dental hook and did the work myself—only more gently. Since then, in addition to daily flossing, I have started brushing my teeth with a drop (or a few) of herbal oils and extracts—and all the plaque has melted away. No hooks and medieval treatment anymore! Here are some of the herbs I use.

- **Tea tree oil.** This is a great plaque-fighting herb. Use one drop, once a day, together with your regular toothpaste. When you feel your plaque is under control, use it less often (about once a week) because one of the concerns with tea tree oil is that it is allergenic, to a degree. (Your dentist or hygenist can evaluate your plaque and gum pockets.)

- **Probiotic.** Either use organic yogurt with cultures or a probiotic powder with water after you brush your teeth. Swish in your mouth for 2 to 3 minutes, then swallow.

- **Oregano, myrrh, neem, and aloe** (the inside gel of the leaf only): These (and other) herbs can be used to brush teeth and gums. Use one herb extract with each brushing of your teeth, and rotate them so that the likelihood of developing an allergy is reduced. You can also buy neem sticks for cleaning teeth—that is how it has been done in India for thousands of years.

The discussion about fluoride is ongoing. I have read tons of scientific papers about it and still cannot make up my mind. It is a toxic substance, and I am against using it indiscriminately in drinking water. But I like it in toothpaste, as many studies have shown that fluoride greatly reduces cavities. When we use the herbs listed above against gum disease, we are also fighting bacteria with toxic compounds (namely herbs)—only we assume (and have studies to back up our assumption) that herbs are gentler on our bodies than the mining by-product fluoride. Also, we know that herbs help fight gum disease, but they are less established against cavities, while probiotics do both.

Eating fresh and fermented food, chewing well, not snacking between meals, and avoiding sugary beverages (including all juices!) will go a long way toward protecting your teeth. Still, you should see a dentist regularly to make sure that little problems don't creep up. A small hole is easily mended, but a big hole might mean that your tooth has to come out.

Urinary Tract Infection (UTI)

Odors often signal that your urine is infected even before you experience burning and the urge to urinate often. So if you notice a strange smell, start working immediately—before the infection gets out of hand!

Most UTIs that are caught early on can be dealt with simply, with herbs, probiotics, and so on. Despite popular belief, antibiotics should be reserved for genuinely dangerous infections. Not only should we curb antibiotic use because of the development of possible antibiotic resistances in bacteria, but we should also curb it because it has been shown that bacteria burrow into the bladder wall during a course of antibiotics, only to pop up again a bit later![30]

Before we discuss natural treatments, I must provide this warning: *Immediately* see your physician or visit the emergency room if you have any of these signs or symptoms.

- Blood in your urine
- Pus from your vagina or penis
- Fever, because *any* fever means that the infection has gone beyond the confines of your bladder
- Flank/kidney pains, because if you have pain that far away from your bladder, it means that the UTI has ascended to your kidneys or that you have kidney stones

Additionally, all children with UTIs as well as any adult who has never had a UTI before should immediately see a doctor.

Other symptoms of a UTI include:

- Cloudy urine
- Strong, offensive odor
- Discomfort, pain, and burning in your bladder area
- The urge to urinate frequently without producing much

A common cause of UTIs, especially in women, is sexual intercourse. Women have a very short urethra, so bacteria can spread easily and invade the bladder. UTIs are most common in young women (who typically have more frequent sex) and in women after menopause (the lack of estrogen leads to shrinking tissues, which means less protection against invading bacteria). But just because you may fall into one of these two groups doesn't mean you're doomed to struggle with UTIs forever. Here are a few tips for preventing UTIs.

- Avoid all sugar and white starches. Eating healthy foods builds up good bowel bacteria, which builds a stronger immune system.
- If you tend to get UTIs often, take cranberry capsules after sexual intercourse. The antioxidants in cranberries prevent bacteria from lodging into the bladder mucosa. If you don't have cranberry supplements on hand, similar proanthocyanidins (a certain group of antioxidants found in cranberries) are also found in blueberries and strongly colored fruits and vegetables, teas (black and green), black currants, bilberries, grape seeds, grape skins, and red wines.
- Drink enough hot fluid each day to flush out bacteria.
- Take a daily probiotic, which helps get rid of bad bacteria in your bowel. (These are most often the culprit in urinary tract infections.)

- Do Kegel exercises, walk regularly, or stand on one leg to strengthen your pelvic muscles. If those muscles are weak, you might not be able to empty your bladder fully each time, and that puts you at an increased risk for recurrent UTIs.

- Regularly take women's herbs like black cohosh and vitex during and after menopause to strengthen your vaginal mucosa.

We all know that prevention is better than treatment. But when, while voiding, you get the familiar sensation of burning that heralds a UTI, you should act quickly; the earlier you catch an infection, the easier it is to treat. If you find that you've developed the symptoms of a UTI despite taking the precautions listed above, try a few of these natural supplements.

- Uva ursi (*Arctostaphylos uva-ursi*)[31] is antimicrobial (killing germs) and anti-inflammatory. Both of these properties come in handy while treating a urinary tract infection.

- *Usnea* spp. This group of lichens that grow on trees is strongly anti-bacterial. *Usnea* should not be taken for longer than a few days because of possible liver toxicity. This has been used widely against urinary tract infections, but no study on people has been done (which is the case for so many good herbal treatments).

- Also worth trying is D-mannose, which is not strictly an herb, but a sugar. It only works against *E. coli*, which happens to be the most commonly found bacterium in UTIs.

Vaginal Infections

As your tissues are bathed in higher levels of glucose than normal, they tend to develop yeast infections that go away with treatment but return rapidly if your blood glucose is not kept down. This problem can cause itching, an unpleasant odor, and discomfort during sex. If you've had a yeast infection before and recognize the signs, you can try to treat it at home. To do this, use a syringe to apply 5 milliliters of plain yogurt into your vagina daily until the symptoms disappear. The yogurt provides lactobacilli, which are needed in the vagina to maintain proper pH balance. In addition to the yogurt, you can also treat a yeast infection with tea tree oil suppositories or probiotic vaginal suppositories, both available at health food stores. More serious infections should be evaluated by your physician.

Varicose Veins

Varicose veins are thought to be ugly, and in a way, they are. But as a doctor, I am less concerned with beauty and more concerned with health problems—and varicose veins are not as harmless as they seem.

Thrombosis is a clot that blocks a vein, usually in one leg, and may lead to pulmonary embolus and, in rare cases, a stroke. Both can be fatal. The symp-

Mother Nature's Miracle Oil

Wouldn't it be great if we had a drug that would work against bacteria, viruses, and fungi? Well, we have that drug, brought to us by Mother Nature: tea tree oil (*Melaleuca alternifolia*). This essential oil from the leaves of a small Australian tree in the myrtle family fights all kinds of germs. (Don't confuse it with "tea oil," which comes in big bottles and is used for cooking. Tea tree oil can only be applied externally. Taken internally, it is toxic and can be fatal.)

This miracle oil is perfect for treating many different skin conditions. Tea tree oil does not usually irritate the skin, but if you experience increased redness after application, the possibility of an allergy needs to be considered; another possibility would be a worsening infection.

Tea tree oil belongs in every first aid kit as an all-around antiseptic. It is anti-inflammatory and has a healing effect on the skin. In small doses, it is said to stimulate the immune system—but this is definitely not a substance I would ingest. Here are some great uses for this versatile oil.

- **Eliminate bacteria.** Infected hangnails, pimples, abrasions, and staphylococcus, even against resistant staph, if the area is not too large. Apply tea tree oil to the problem area as needed, several times a day. With large wounds, there is the danger of absorption and internal toxicity, so avoid tea tree oil and instead use neem oil.

- **Improve acne.** Place five drops of tea tree oil on a moist facecloth and rub your skin gently, avoiding your eyes. Do this once a day. (You can also use undiluted tea tree oil on blackheads and whiteheads to make them disappear.)

toms are swelling, pain, and warmth in the affected limb. Physicians order a Doppler scan to determine whether the patient has a clot. If a clot is present, the patient will be admitted to a hospital and heparin, warfarin (Coumadin), and other anticoagulants will be used to thin the blood until the clot is gone or at least stabilized.

The good news is that the Doppler test often comes back negative. Typical findings are that the patient "only" has phlebitis, an inflammation of the wall

- **Fight viruses.** Apply tea tree oil to cold sores, warts, chickenpox, and shingles to reduce your recovery time.

- **Kill bugs.** You can fight lice by rubbing your scalp with tea tree oil or scabies by applying the oil to affected areas.

- **Stop itching.** Try tea tree oil on minor itches. For insect bites, place a drop on the itchy or painful area to eliminate itching and begin the healing process.

- **Soothe a sore throat.** Add one drop of tea tree oil to one glass of water. Gargle for a few seconds, but don't swallow, to find relief. (This also works to freshen breath and fight gingivitis and periodontitis.)

- **Relieve pain.** Tea tree oil is especially helpful for treating the pain of mild burns and sunburns. Just apply a small amount to the area that's causing pain. Repeat as needed.

- **Reduce dandruff** Add a few drops of tea tree oil to your shampoo.

- **Relieve sweaty, smelly feet.** Apply a few drops of tea tree oil to your feet after washing them with soap.

- **Aromatherapy.** A tiny drop goes a very long way. Thought to be a balm for the soul, tea tree oil is believed to have healing properties for psychological traumas and to help fight anxiety, increase confidence, and help when one is exhausted and discouraged. Some migraine sufferers are helped by smelling tea tree oil in the air.

of a vein. The symptoms are exactly the same: pain, swelling, and warmth. So what can you do for inflamed veins? Phlebitis and thrombosis can have several causes, and sometimes it's a combination: A genetic disposition plays a role. Longtime immobility—like sitting during a long flight without getting up, or being bed-ridden, especially after surgery—is known to cause clots. Hormone therapy can also lead to clotting. Less well-known reasons

Singing the Praises of Aloe Vera

Even if you have a black thumb and all plants wither if you just look at them, you should still have one houseplant: aloe vera. It doesn't take much effort to care for it—just put it on a windowsill and water it once in a while. The danger is more in overwatering, not in underwatering, as it is a desert plant. You can also buy huge aloe leaves in Chinese supermarkets and local health food stores; just make sure to wash them with a mild detergent to remove pesticides before using them!

Aloe vera is a succulent (meaning water-storing) plant that comes from the arid regions of the Arabic peninsula and Northern Africa. It has been cultivated for thousands of years due to its medicinal properties, and you can no longer find any natural stands in the wild—all existing plants seem to have been planted purposefully, which is certainly a hint of its usefulness. Aloe has long, leathery leaves with little spines or hooks along the edges. The leaves can be spotted or not, and the plant can be small or large. Regardless of its size, though, all aloes seem to work—but aloe vera is the one that has been studied extensively.

So why do I want to sing the praises of aloe vera here? Last week, while concentrating on my Chinese calligraphy, admiring the black lines of my brush on the paper, suddenly a beautiful red streak mixed itself in, creating a truly amazing color scheme: black, white, and bright red. Only, the red was bleeding from one of my knuckles—and I didn't even know how I had hurt myself. A flap of skin was barely hanging on. I applied a bit of tea tree oil and a bandage, and I continued with my calligraphy. It healed slowly (being on the knuckle, where constant movement stretches the skin, didn't help). Every time I thought I could take off the bandage, the flap stuck to it, and the wound ripped open and bled again.

are cancer and food sensitivities, or even just eating inflammatory food.

As you now know, poor nutrition promotes inflammation, and the list of diseases linked to inflammation is growing. Phlebitis and thrombosis are two of them. Junk foods with a high sugar content, white starches, trans fats, and dairy are highly inflammatory for everyone. Food sensitivities, on the other hand, can also inflame. But the causative foods are sometimes hard to

Then I thought of aloe. I have several plants in the house, so I cut off one of the fleshy leaves at the base and dripped some of its juice onto my knuckle after I had reapplied tea tree oil. Aloe vera is said to have antiseptic properties as well, but tea tree oil is always my first choice to prevent infection in wounds. This time, I skipped the bandage. Within minutes of applying the aloe juice, the wound looked less angry. After 2 hours, it had shrunk to about half its size. I could now see what was still viable tissue and what was not, so I cut off the dead skin, and now I am not as likely to rip open the wound again.

In addition to soothing your skin, you may also use aloe vera for the following purposes.

- **Wound healing, including burns.** *Note:* Because aloe heals wounds so quickly, it should never be applied to a deep wound—say, a bedsore, a surgical cut, or a deep diabetic ulcer. Aloe would speed up superficial healing and wound closure, but the underlying wound could still be smoldering, putting it at risk to break open again.

- **Gum healing.** Include a small drop of the gel with your toothpaste before you brush or just chew a piece of the gel.

- **Stomach-soothing.** Aloe is especially good against heartburn and ulcers. (Eat a small amount of the gel to reap these benefits.)

- **Softening and smoothing the skin.** It's especially useful in providing relief from eczema.

Aloe vera serves many purposes; you can probably find even more uses. But its healing powers alone should bring it into every household!

pinpoint, as they vary from person to person. I have seen allergic reactions to gluten, bananas, avocados, nuts, beef (it might be more what the cattle ate than the beef itself), and cherries—but the possibilities are endless; a food diary might help you determine the cause, in recurrent cases.

Varicose veins are one of the signs of inflamation in the body. Slowly, over the years, the varicosities grow, which is often thought of as being just another sign of aging. Pregnancies and prolonged standing can also aggravate the condition.

If you find your varicose veins particularly troublesome, follow the tips below to reduce their discomfort and severity.

- Go on a search for offending foods and eliminate them.
- Move your body moderately. (Don't sit for long periods, and go for a walk every day.)
- Don't sit with your legs crossed, which clamps down the bloodflow.
- Elevate your legs as often as possible.
- Take high-dosage fish oil supplements (2,000 milligrams per day). Be sure to discuss this with your doctor, though, because in addition to being anti-inflammatory, fish oil is a mild blood thinner and could be contraindicated with some conditions.
- Whether it's a cold shower, sitz bath, or even a walk in the ocean, applying cold water to your legs is very beneficial and brings instant relief.
- If your situation is acute, applying an icepack for no longer than 15 minutes at a time might bring relief.
- Wear support hose or tights at all times, even in summer. They prevent the veins from bulging out and growing bigger and bigger. Continue to wear the support hose after you are better to prevent recurrence. Regular support panty hose are less tedious than medical stockings, which also have a tendency to cut off bloodflow at the cuff—exactly what should be avoided.
- Don't rush into surgery. Phlebitis is not just a mechanical problem, like a poorly functioning valve. Consider a food connection first.
- If your symptoms don't improve with these methods, return to your physician—soon! One dreaded consequence of a leg clot is tiny emboli traveling to the lungs, which can be fatal.

ENDNOTES

PREFACE
[1] Kim JK, "Inflammation and Insulin Resistance: An Old Story with New Ideas," *Korean Diabetes J.* 34, no. 3 (June 2010): 137–45, published online June 30, 2010.

CHAPTER 1
[1] Wang X et al., "Inflammatory Markers and Risk of Type 2 Diabetes: A Systematic Review and Meta-Analysis," *Diabetes Care* 36, no. 1 (January 2013): 166–75.

[2] Pradhan AD, et al. C-reactive protein, interleukin 6, and risk of developing type 2 diabetes mellitus. *JAMA.* 2001 Jul 18;286(3): 327–34.

[3] Stiles L, Shirihai OS, "Mitochondrial Dynamics and Morphology in Beta-Cells," *Best Pract Res Clin Endocrinol Metab.* 26, no. 6 (December 2012): 725–38, epub July 26, 2012.

[4] Drong AW, Lindgren CM, McCarthy MI, "The Genetic and Epigenetic Basis of Type 2 Diabetes and Obesity," *Clin Pharmacol Ther.* 92, no. 6 (December 2012): 707–15, epub October 10, 2012.

[5] Ling C, Groop L, "Epigenetics: A Molecular Link between Environmental Factors and Type 2 Diabetes," *Diabetes* 58, no. 12 (December 2009): 2718–25.

[6] Camilleri M, "Mechanisms of Disease: Peripheral Mechanisms in Irritable Bowel Syndrome," *NEJM* 367, no. 17 (October 25, 2012): 1626–35.

CHAPTER 2
[1] Gallagher EJ, LeRoith D, "The Proliferating Role of Insulin and Insulin-Like Growth Factors in Cancer," *Trends Endocrinol Metab,* 21, no. 10 (October 2010): 610–18, published online July 19, 2010.

[2] Brown RJ et al., "Uncoupling Intensive Insulin Therapy from Weight Gain and Hypoglycemia in Type 1 Diabetes," *Diabetes Technol Ther.* 13, no. 4 (April 2011): 457–60.

[3] Williams JW et al., "Preventing Alzheimer's Disease and Cognitive Decline," *Evidence Reports/Technology Assessments,* no. 193.

[4] Shelton RC, Miller AH, "Eating Ourselves to Death and Despair: The Contribution of Adiposity and Inflammation to Depression," *Prog Neurobiol.* 91, no. 4 (August 2010): 275–99, published online April 22, 2010.

[5] Fernandez-Egea E et al., "Parental History of Type 2 Diabetes in Patients with Nonaffective Psychosis," *Schizophr Res.* 98, no. 1–3 (January 2008): 302–6, epub November 26, 2007.

[6] Petrofsky JS, "The Effect of Type-2-Diabetes-Related Vascular Endothelial Dysfunction on Skin Physiology and Activities of Daily Living," *J Diabetes Sci Technol.* 5, no. 3 (May 2011): 657–667, published online May 1, 2011.

[7] Preshaw PM et al., "Periodontitis and Diabetes: A Two-Way Relationship," *Diabetologia* 55, no. 1 (January 2012): 21–31, published online November 6, 2011.

[8] Mojarad F, Maybodi MH, "Association Between Dental Caries and Body Mass Index Among Hamedan Elementary School Children in 2009," *J Dent (Tehran)* 8, no. 4 (Autumn 2011): 170–77, published online December 20, 2011

[9] Mirrakhimov AE, "Chronic Obstructive Pulmonary Disease and Glucose Metabolism: A Bitter Sweet Symphony," *Cardiovasc Diabetol.* 11 (2012): 132, published online October 27, 2012.

[10] Flores-Le Roux JA et al., "Seven-Year Mortality in Heart Failure Patients with Undiagnosed Diabetes: An Observational Study," *Cardiovasc Diabetol.* 10 (2011): 39, published online May 4, 2011.

[11] Abdulameer SA et al., "Osteoporosis and Type 2 Diabetes Mellitus: What Do We Know, and What We Can Do?" *Patient Prefer Adherence* 6 (2012): 435–48, published online June 11, 2012.

[12] Choung RS et al., "Risk of Gastroparesis in Subjects with Type 1 and 2 Diabetes in the General Population," *Am J Gastroenterol.* 107, no. 1 (January 2012): 82–88, published online November 15, 2011.

[13] Lee SD et al., "Gastroesophageal Reflux Disease in Type II Diabetes Mellitus With or Without Peripheral Neuropathy," *J Neurogastroenterol Motil.* 2011 July; 17(3): 274–78, published online July 14, 2011.

[14] Hatziagelaki E et al., "Predictors of Impaired Glucose Regulation in Patients with Non-Alcoholic Fatty Liver Disease," *Exp Diabetes Res.* (2012): 351974, published online September 21, 2011.

[15] van der Meer V et al., "Chronic Kidney Disease in Patients with Diabetes Mellitus Type 2 or Hypertension in General Practice," *Br J Gen Pract.* 60, no. 581 (December 1, 2010): 884–90.

[16] Romano-Keeler J, Weitkamp J-H, Moore DJ, "Regulatory Properties of the Intestinal Microbiome Effecting the Development and Treatment of Diabetes," *Curr Opin Endocrinol Diabetes Obes.* 19, no. 2 (April 2012): 73–80.

[17] Li D, "Diabetes and Pancreatic Cancer," *Mol Carcinog.* 51, no. 1 (January 2012): 64–74.

[18] Gouveri E, Papanas N, Maltezos E, "The Female Breast and Diabetes," *Breast* 20, no. 3 (June 2011): 205–11, epub March 16, 2011.

[19] Zhiqin Bu Z et al., "The Relationship Between Polycystic Ovary Syndrome, Glucose Tolerance Status and Serum Preptin Level," *Reprod Biol Endocrinol.* 10 (2012): 10, published online February 6, 2012.

[20] Saad F, Gooren LJ, "The Role of Testosterone in the Etiology and Treatment of Obesity, the Metabolic Syndrome, and Diabetes Mellitus Type 2," *J Obes.* 2011 (2011): 471584, published online August 10, 2010.

[21] Sharifi F et al., "Independent Predictors of Erectile Dysfunction in Type 2 Diabetes Mellitus: Is It True What They Say about Risk Factors?" *ISRN Endocrinol.* 2012 (2012): 502353, published online August 27, 2012.

[22] Rowe BR et al., "Is Candidiasis the True Cause of Vulvovaginal Irritation in Women with Diabetes Mellitus?" *J Clin Pathol.* 43, no. 8 (August 1990): 644–45.

[23] Mazhar K et al., "Severity of Diabetic Retinopathy and Health-Related Quality of Life: The Los Angeles Latino Eye Study," *Ophthalmology* 118, no. 4 (April 2011): 649–55, published online October 29, 2010.

[24] Frisina ST et al., "Characterization of Hearing Loss in Aged Type II Diabetics," *Hear Res.* 211, no. 1–2 (January 2006): 103–13, published online November 23, 2005.

[25] Little TJ, Feinle-Bisset C, "Oral and Gastrointestinal Sensing of Dietary Fat and Appetite Regulation in Humans: Modification by Diet and Obesity," *Front Neurosci.* 4 (2010): 178, published online October 19, 2010, prepublished online May 20, 2010.

[26] Jackson RM, Rice DH, "Acute Bacterial Sinusitis and Diabetes Mellitus," *Otolaryngol Head Neck Surg.* 97, no. 5 (November 1987): 469–73.

[27] LeBrasseur NK, Walsh K, Arany Z, "Metabolic Benefits of Resistance Training and Fast Glycolytic Skeletal Muscle," *Am J Physiol Endocrinol Metab.* 300, no. 1 (January 2011): E3–E10, published online November 2, 2010.

[28] Rosenbloom AL, Silverstein JH, "Connective Tissue and Joint Disease in Diabetes Mellitus," *Endocrinol Metab Clin North Am.* 25, no. 2 (June 1996): 473–83.

[29] Wen-Sheng Yue W-S et al., "Impact of Glycemic Control on Circulating Endothelial Progenitor Cells and Arterial Stiffness in Patients with Type 2 Diabetes Mellitus," *Cardiovasc Diabetol.* 10 (2011): 113, published online December 20, 2011.

[30] Stegenga ME et al., "Hyperglycemia Enhances Coagulation and Reduces Neutrophil Degranulation, Whereas Hyperinsulinemia Inhibits Fibrinolysis During Human Endotoxemia," *Blood* 112, no. 1 (July 1, 2008): 82–89, prepublished online March 3, 2008.

[31] Garces-Sanchez M et al., "Painless Diabetic Motor Neuropathy: A Variant of DLRPN?" *Ann Neurol.* 69, no. 6 (June 2011): 1043–54, published online March 18, 2011.

[32] Chakraborty S et al., "Lymphatic System Acts as a Vital Link between Metabolic Syndrome and Inflammation," *Ann N Y Acad Sci.* 1207, suppl. 1 (October 2010): E94–102.

[33] Paspala I et al., "The Role of Psychobiological and Neuroendocrine Mechanisms in Appetite Regulation and Obesity," *Open Cardiovasc Med J.* 6 (2012): 147–55, published online December 28, 2012.

[34] Bankoski A et al., "Sedentary Activity Associated with Metabolic Syndrome Independent of Physical Activity," *Diabetes Care.* 34, no. 2 (February 2011): 497–503, published online January 20, 2011.

[35] Darin E, Olson DE et al., "Screening for Diabetes and Pre-Diabetes With Proposed A1c-Based Diagnostic Criteria," *Diabetes Care.* 33, no. 10 (October 2010): 2184–89, published online July 16, 2010.

[36] Raz I et al., "Diabetes: Insulin Resistance and Derangements in Lipid Metabolism. Cure through Intervention in Fat Transport and Storage," *Diabetes Metab Res Rev.* 21, no. 1 (Jan–Feb 2005): 3–14.

[37] Bagi Z, Feher A, Cassuto J, "Microvascular Responsiveness in Obesity: Implications for Therapeutic Intervention," *Br J Pharmacol.* 165, no. 3 (February 2012): 544–60.

[38] Patti M-E, Corvera S, "The Role of Mitochondria in the Pathogenesis of Type 2 Diabetes," *Endocr Rev.* 31, no. 3 (June 2010): 364–95, published online February 15, 2010.

[39] Shapiro H, Lutaty A, Ariel A, "Macrophages, Meta-Inflammation, and Immuno-Metabolism," *ScientificWorldJournal.* 11 (2011): 2509–29, published online December 28, 2011.

[40] Nakagawa T et al., "A Causal Role for Uric Acid in Fructose-Induced Metabolic Syndrome," *Am J Physiol Renal Physiol.* 290, no. 3 (March 2006): F625–31, first published October 18, 2005.

[41] Paspala I et al., "The Role of Psychobiological and Neuroendocrine Mechanisms in Appetite Regulation and Obesity," *Open Cardiovasc Med J.* 6 (2012): 147–55, published online December 28, 2012.

[42] Roberts DC, "Quick Weight Loss: Sorting Fad from Fact," *Med J Aust.* 175, no. 11–12 (December 3–17, 2001): 637–40.

[43] Willis BL et al., "Midlife Fitness and the Development of Chronic Conditions in Later Life," *Arch Intern Med.* 172, no. 17 (2012): 1–8.

[44] Carnethon MR et al., "Association of Weight Status with Mortality in Adults with Incident Diabetes," *JAMA* 308, no. 6 (August 8, 2012): 581–90.

[45] Sánchez JC et al., "Celiac Disease Associated Antibodies in Persons with Latent Autoimmune Diabetes of Adult and Type 2 Diabetes," *Autoimmunity* 40, no. 2 (March 2007): 103–7.

[46] Catassi C, "The Global Village of Celiac Disease," [article in Italian] *Recenti Prog Med.* 92, no. 7–8 (July–August 2001): 446–50.

[47] Rubio-Tapia A et al., "Increased Prevalence and Mortality in Undiagnosed Celiac Disease," *Gastroenterology* 137, no. 1 (July 2009): 88–93, published online April 10, 2009.

CHAPTER 3

[1] International Diabetes Federation Web site: http://www.idf.org/diabetesatlas/5e/ Update2012 (accessed January 12, 2013).

[2] International Diabetes Federation, *Diabetes Atlas 2012 Update.*

[3] Petersen M, for American Diabetes Association, "Economic Costs of Diabetes in the US in 2007," *Diabetes Care* 31, no. 3 (March 2008): 596–615.

[4] Diabetes Statistics, data from the 2011 *National Diabetes Fact Sheet* (released January 26, 2011), accessed January 12, 2013, on: http://www.diabetes.org/diabetes-basics/diabetes-statistics/.

[5] Ogden CL et al., "Prevalence and Trends in Overweight Among US Children and Adolescents, 1999–2000," *JAMA* 288, no. 14 (October 9, 2002): 1728–32.

[6] Wei W et al., "A Clinical Study on the Short-Term Effect of Berberine in Comparison to Metformin on the Metabolic Characteristics of Women with Polycystic Ovary Syndrome," *Eur J Endocrinol.* 166, no. 1 (January 2012): 99–105.

[7] Yin J et al., "Berberine Improves Glucose Metabolism through Induction of Glycolysis," *Am J Physiol Endocrinol Metab.* 294, no. 1 (January 2008): E148–56.

[8] Tan W et al., "Berberine Hydrochloride: Anticancer Activity and Nanoparticulate Delivery System," *Int J Nanomed.* 6 (2011): 1773–77.

[9] See note 6 above.

[10] Boussageon R et al., "Reappraisal of Metformin Efficacy in the Treatment of Type 2 Diabetes: A Meta-Analysis of Randomised Controlled Trials," *PLOS Medicine*, April 2012.

[11] Reasner C et al., "The Effect of Initial Therapy with the Fixed-Dose Combination of Sitagliptin and Metformin Compared with Metformin Monotherapy in Patients with Type 2 Diabetes Mellitus," *Diabetes Obes Metab.* 13, no. 7 (July 2011): 644–52.

[12] Fu AZ et al., "Initial Sulfonylurea Use and Subsequent Insulin Therapy in Older

Subjects with Type 2 Diabetes Mellitus," *Diabetes Ther.* 3, no. 1 (November 2012): 12, epub October 18, 2012.

[13] Gallwitz B et al., "2-Year Efficacy and Safety of Linagliptin Compared with Glimepiride in Patients with Type 2 Diabetes Inadequately Controlled on Metformin: A Randomised, Double-Blind, Non-Inferiority Trial," *Lancet* 380, no. 9840 (August 4, 2012): 475–83, epub June 28, 2012.

[14] Gram J et al., "Pharmacological Treatment of the Pathogenetic Defects in Type 2 Diabetes. The Randomized Multicenter South Danish Diabetes Study," *Diabetes Care* 34, no. 1 (January 2011): 27–33, published online October 7, 2010.

[15] www.mayoclinic.com/health/insulin-and-weight-gain/DA00139, accessed January 18, 2013.

[16] Rodin J, "Insulin Levels, Hunger, and Food Intake: An Example of Feedback Loops in Body Weight Regulation," *Health Psychol.* 4, no. 1 (1985): 1–24.

[17] Heinemann L, "Hypoglycemia and Insulin Analogues: Is There a Reduction in the Incidence?" *J Diabetes Complications* 13, no. 2 (Mar–Apr 1999): 105–14.

[18] Psaltopoulou T, Ilias I, Alevizaki M, "The Role of Diet and Lifestyle in Primary, Secondary, and Tertiary Diabetes Prevention: A Review of Meta-Analyses," *Rev Diabet Stud.* 7, no. 1 (Spring 2010): 26–35, published online May 10, 2010.

[19] Li GW et al., "The Long-Term Effect of Lifestyle Interventions to Prevent Diabetes in the China Da Qing Diabetes Prevention Study: A 20-Year Follow-Up Study," *The Lancet* 371, no. 9626 (May 24, 2008): 1783–89.

[20] Sun G, Kashyap SR, "Cancer Risk in Type 2 Diabetes Mellitus: Metabolic Links and Therapeutic Considerations," *J Nutr Metab.* 2011: 708183, published online June 1, 2011.

[21] Kornaat PR et al., "Positive Association between Increased Popliteal Artery Vessel Wall Thickness and Generalized Osteoarthritis: Is OA Also Part of the Metabolic Syndrome?" *Skeletal Radiol.* 38, no. 12 (December 2009): 1147–51, published online July 3, 2009.

[22] Naranjo DM et al., "Patients with Type 2 Diabetes at Risk for Major Depressive Disorder Over Time," *Ann Fam Med.* 9, no. 2 (March 2011): 115–20.

[23] Kawser Akter K et al., "Diabetes Mellitus and Alzheimer's Disease: Shared Pathology and Treatment?" *Br J Clin Pharmacol.* 71, no. 3 (March 2011): 365–76.

[24] van Dijk H et al., "Early Neurodegeneration in the Retina of Type 2 Diabetic Patients," *Invest Ophthalmol Vis Sci.* 53, no. 6 (May 2012): 2715–19, published online May 14, 2012.

[25] Aziz Z et al., "Predictive Factors for Lower Extremity Amputations in Diabetic Foot Infections," *Diabet Foot Ankle*, published online September 20, 2011.

[26] Yamada T et al., "Erectile Dysfunction and Cardiovascular Events in Diabetic Men: A Meta-Analysis of Observational Studies," *PLoS One* 7, no. 9 (2012): e43673, published online September 4, 2012.

[27] Bakris GL, "Recognition, Pathogenesis, and Treatment of Different Stages of Nephropathy in Patients with Type 2 Diabetes Mellitus," *Mayo Clin Proc.* 86, no. 5 (May 2011): 444–56.

[28] Nelson SM, Matthews P, Poston L, "Maternal Metabolism and Obesity: Modifiable Determinants of Pregnancy Outcome," *Hum Reprod Update* 16, no. 3 (May–June 2010): 255–75, published online December 4, 2009.

[29] Keymel S, "Characterization of Macro- and Microvascular Function and Structure in Patients with Type 2 Diabetes Mellitus," *Am J Cardiovasc Dis.* 1, no. 1 (2011): 68–75, published online May 15, 2011.

[30] Casqueiro J, Casqueiro J, Alves C, "Infections in Patients with Diabetes Mellitus: A Review of Pathogenesis," *Indian J Endocrinol Metab.* 16, suppl. 1 (March 2012): S27–S36.

[31] Hammar N et al., "Incidence of Urinary Tract Infection in Patients with Type 2 Diabetes. Experience from Adverse Event Reporting in Clinical Trials," *Pharmacoepidemiol Drug Saf.* 19, no. 12 (December 2010): 1287–92, epub October 21, 2010.

[32] El-Gilany AH, Fathy H, "Risk Factors of Recurrent Furunculosis," *Dermatol Online J.* 15, no. 1 (January 15, 2009): 16.

[33] Márquez Balbás G, Sánchez Regaña M, Millet PU, "Study on the Use of Omega-3 Fatty Acids as a Therapeutic Supplement in Treatment of Psoriasis," *Clin Cosmet Investig Dermatol.* 4 (2011): 73–77, published online June 20, 2011.

[34] Rosen ED, Spiegelman BM, "Adipocytes as Regulators of Energy Balance and Glucose Homeostasis," *Nature* 444, no. 7121 (December 14, 2006): 847–53.

[35] Hernández C et al., "Effect of Intensive Insulin Therapy on Macular Biometrics, Plasma VEGF and Its Soluble Receptor in Newly Diagnosed Diabetic Patients," *Diabetes Metab Res Rev.* 26, no. 5 (July 2010): 386–92.

[36] Gurav AN, "Periodontal Therapy: An Adjuvant for Glycemic Control," *Diabetes Metab Syndr.* 6, no. 4 (October 2012): 218–23, epub October 24, 2012.

[37] Chanussot C, Arenas R, "Interdigital and Foot Fungal Infection in Patients with Onychomycosis" [article in Spanish], *Rev Iberoam Micol.* 24, no. 2 (June 2007): 118–21.

[39] de Leon EM et al., "Prevalence and Risk Factors for Vaginal *Candida* Colonization in Women with Type 1 and Type 2 Diabetes," *BMC Infect Dis.* 2 (2002): 1, epub January 30, 2002.

[39] Choung RS et al., "Risk of Gastroparesis in Subjects with Type 1 and 2 Diabetes in the General Population," *Am J Gastroenterol.* 107, no. 1 (January 2012): 82–88, epub November 15, 2011.

[40] Al-Matubsi HY et al., "Diabetic Hand Syndromes as a Clinical and Diagnostic Tool for Diabetes Mellitus Patients," *Diabetes Res Clin Pract.* 94, no. 2 (November 2011): 225–29, epub August 9, 2011.

[41] Seftel AD et al., "Advanced Glycation End Products in Human Penis: Elevation in Diabetic Tissue, Site of Deposition, and Possible Effect through iNOS or eNOS," *Urology* 50, no. 6 (December 1997): 1016–26.

CHAPTER 4

[1] Menshikova EV et al., "Deficiency of Subsarcolemmal Mitochondria in Obesity and Type 2 Diabetes," *Diabetes* 54, no. 1 (January 2005): 8–14.

[2] Dela F, Helge JW, "Insulin Resistance and Mitochondrial Function in Skeletal Muscle," *Int J Biochem Cell Biol.* 45, no. 1 (January 2013): 11–15, epub October 2, 2012.

[3] Champaneri S et al., "Biological Basis of Depression in Adults with Diabetes," *Curr Diab Rep.* 10, no. 6 (December 2010): 396–405.

[4] Anisman H, Hayley S, "Inflammatory Factors Contribute to Depression and Its Comorbid Conditions," *Sci Signal.* 5, no. 244 (October 2, 2012): pe45.

CHAPTER 5

[1] Simmons RK, et al., "Screening for Type 2 Diabetes and Population Mortality over 10 Years (ADDITION-Cambridge): A Cluster-Randomised Controlled Trial," *The Lancet* 380, no. 9855 (November 2012): 1741–48.

[2] Dulloo AG, Montani JP, "Body Composition, Inflammation and Thermogenesis in Pathways to Obesity and the Metabolic Syndrome: An Overview," *Obes Rev.* suppl. 2 (December 13, 2012): 1–5.

[3] Carnethon MR et al., "Association of Weight Status with Mortality in Adults with Incident Diabetes," *JAMA* 308, no. 6 (August 8, 2012): 581–90.

[4] Lovell-Smith D, Kenealy T, Buetow S, "Eating When Empty Is Good for Your Health," *Med Hypotheses.* 75, no. 2 (August 2010): 172–78, epub March 15, 2010.

[5] Schneeberger M, Claret M, "Recent Insights into the Role of Hypothalamic AMPK Signaling Cascade upon Metabolic Control," *Front Neurosci.* 6 (2012): 185, epub December 20, 2012.

[6] Ayus JC, Arieff AI, "Abnormalities of Water Metabolism in the Elderly," *Semin Nephrol.* 16, no. 4 (July 1996): 277–88.

[7] Story M, French S, "Food Advertising and Marketing Directed at Children and Adolescents in the US," *International Journal of Behavioral Nutrition and Physical Activity* 1 (2004): 3.

[8] Mennella JA et al., "Prenatal and Postnatal Flavor Learning by Human Infants," *Pediatrics* 107, no. 6 (June 1, 2001): e88.

[9] Skinner MK, "Metabolic Disorders: Fathers' Nutritional Legacy," *Nature.* 467, no. 7318 (October 21, 2010): 922–23.

[10] Schiavo-Cardozo D, "Appetite-Regulating Hormones from the Upper Gut: Disrupted Control of Xenin and Ghrelin in Night Workers," *Clin Endocrinol (Oxf).* December 1, 2012, epub ahead of print.

[11] Leeuwen WMA van et al., "Sleep Restriction Affects Glucose Metabolism in Healthy Young Men," *International Journal of Endocrinology,* 2010 (2010): article ID 108641.

[12] Spiegel K, "Twenty-Four-Hour Profiles of Acylated and Total Ghrelin: Relationship with Glucose Levels and Impact of Time of Day and Sleep," *J Clin Endocrinol Metab.* 96, no. 2 (February 2011): 486–493.

[13] Cho H, Zhao X, Hatori M, et al., "Regulation of Circadian Behaviour and Metabolism by REV-ERB-α and REV-ERB-β," *Nature* 485, no. 7396 (March 29, 2012):123–7.

[14] Mason C et al., "History of Weight Cycling Does Not Impede Future Weight Loss or Metabolic Improvements in Postmenopausal Women," *Metabolism,* published online August 14, 2012.

[15] Davis C et al., "Binge Eating Disorder and the Dopamine D2 Receptor: Genotypes and Sub-phenotypes," *Prog Neuropsychopharmacol Biol Psychiatry.* 38, no. 2 (August 7, 2012): 328–35, epub May 8, 2012.

[16] Liu Z, Li N, Neu J, "Tight Junctions, Leaky Intestines, and Pediatric Diseases," *Acta Paediatr.* 94, no. 4 (April 2005): 386–93.

[17] Drisko J et al., "Treating Irritable Bowel Syndrome with a Food Elimination Diet Followed by Food Challenge and Probiotics," *J Am Coll Nutr.* 25, no. 6 (December 2006): 514–22.

[18] Islam SA, Luster AD, "T Cell Homing to Epithelial Barriers in Allergic Disease," *Nat Med.* 18, no. 5 (May 4, 2012): 705–15.

[19] Keller H et al., "Issues Associated with the Use of Modified Texture Foods," *J Nutr Health Aging.* 16, no. 3 (March 2012): 195–200.

[20] Holt RR, "The Potential of Flavanol and Procyanidin Intake to Influence Age-Related Vascular Disease," *J Nutr Gerontol Geriatr.* 32, no. 3 (2012): 290–323.

[21] Shoham DA et al., "An Actor-Based Model of Social Network Influence on Adolescent Body Size, Screen Time, and Playing Sports," *PLoS One.* 7, no. 6 (2012): e39795, published online June 29, 2012.

[22] MacLean PS et al., "Biology's Response to Dieting: The Impetus for Weight Regain," *Am J Physiol Regul Integr Comp Physiol.* 301, no. 3 (September 2011): R581–R600, published online June 15, 2011.

[23] Li F et al., "Human Gut Bacterial Communities Are Altered by Addition of Cruciferous Vegetables to a Controlled Fruit- and Vegetable-Free Diet," *J Nutr.* 139, no. 9 (September 2009): 1685–91.

[24] Hakansson A, Molin G, "Gut Microbiota and Inflammation," *Nutrients* 3, no. 6 (June 2011): 637–82, published online June 3, 2011.

[25] Resnick C, "Nutritional Protocol for the Treatment of Intestinal Permeability Defects and Related Conditions," *Natural Medicine Journal*, March 1, 2010.

[26] Odegaard J, Chawla A, "Fat's Immune Sentinels," *The Scientist*, December 1, 2012.

[27] Trayhurn P, Wood IS, "Adipokines: Inflammation and the Pleiotropic Role of White Adipose Tissue," *Br J Nutr.* 92, no. 3 (September 2004): 347–55.

[28] Nedergaard J, Becker W, Cannon B, "Effects of Dietary Essential Fatty Acids on Active Thermogenin Content in Rat Brown Adipose Tissue," *The Journal of Nutrition* 113, no. 9 (1983): 1717–24.

[29] Dangardt F et al., "High Physiological Omega-3 Fatty Acid Supplementation Affects Muscle Fatty Acid Composition and Glucose and Insulin Homeostasis in Obese Adolescents," *J Nutr Metab.* (2012): 395757, published online February 20, 2012.

[30] Rosen, ED, Spiegelman BM, "Adipocytes as Regulators of Energy Balance and Glucose Homeostasis," *Nature* 444, no. 7121 (December 14, 2006): 847–53.

[31] Lihn AS, Pedersen SB, Richelsen B, "Adiponectin: Action, Regulation and Association to Insulin Sensitivity," *Obes Rev.* 6, no. 1 (February 2005): 13–21.

[32] Neuhofer A et al., "Impaired Local Production of Pro-Resolving Lipid Mediators in Obesity and 17-HDHA as a Potential Treatment for Obesity-Associated Inflammation," *Diabetes* January 24, 2013, epub ahead of print.

[33] Ding G et al., "Adiponectin and Its Receptors Are Expressed in Adult Ventricular Cardiomyocytes and Upregulated by Activation of Peroxisome Proliferator-Activated Receptor Gamma," *J Mol Cell Cardiol* 43 (2007): 73–84.

[34] Morselli L et al., "Role of Sleep Duration in the Regulation of Glucose Metabolism and Appetite," *Best Pract Res Clin Endocrinol Metab.* 24, no. 5 (October 2010): 687–702.

[35] Corbalán-Tutau D et al., "Daily Profile in Two Circadian Markers 'Melatonin and Cortisol' and Associations with Metabolic Syndrome Components," *Physiol Behav.* June 15, 2012, epub ahead of print.

[36] Zuo H et al., "Association between Serum Leptin Concentrations and Insulin Resistance: A Population-Based Study from China," *PLoS ONE* 8, no. 1 (2013): e54615, epub January 22, 2013.

[37] Boer-Martins L et al., "Relationship of Autonomic Imbalance and Circadian Disruption with Obesity and Type 2 Diabetes in Resistant Hypertensive Patients," *Cardiovasc Diabetol.* 10 (2011): 24, published online March 22, 2011.

[38] Uebaba K et al., "Psychoneuroimmunologic Effects of Ayurvedic Oil-Dripping Treatment," *J Altern Complement Med.* 14, no. 10 (December 2008): 1189–98.

[39] Stafford LD, Welbeck K, "High Hunger State Increases Olfactory Sensitivity to Neutral but Not Food Odors," *Chem Senses.* 36, no. 2 (January 2011): 189–98, epub October 26, 2010.

[40] Castracane VD et al., "Serum Leptin Concentration in Females: Effect of Age, Obesity, and Estrogen Administration," *Fertil Steril* 70 (1998): 472–77.

[41] Meyer MR et al., "Obesity, Insulin Resistance, and Diabetes: Sex Differences and Role of Estrogen Receptors," *Acta Physiol (Oxf).* 203, no. 1 (September 2011): 259–269, published online February 1, 2011.

[42] Richardson AE et al., "Insulin-Like Growth Factor-2 (IGF-2) Activates Estrogen Receptor-α and -β via the IGF-1 and the Insulin Receptors in Breast Cancer Cells," *Growth Factors* 29, no. 2–3 (April 2011): 82–93, published online March 16, 2011.

[43] Mantzoros CS et al., "Leptin in Human Physiology and Pathophysiology," *Am J Physiol Endocrinol Metab.* 301, no. 4 (October 2011): E567–84, published online July 26, 2011.

[44] Lim S et al., "Chronic Exposure to the Herbicide, Atrazine, Causes Mitochondrial Dysfunction and Insulin Resistance," *PLoS One*, no. 4: e5186.

[45] Spreadbury I, "Comparison with Ancestral Diets Suggests Dense Acellular Carbohydrates Promote an Inflammatory Microbiota, and May Be the Primary Dietary Cause of Leptin Resistance and Obesity," *Diabetes Metab Syndr Obes.* 5 (2012): 175–89, published online July 6, 2012.

[46] Siri-Tarino PW, "Saturated Fat, Carbohydrate, and Cardiovascular Disease," *Am J Clin Nutr.* 91, no. 3 (March 2010): 502–9, published online January 20, 2010.

[47] Zadoks RN et al., "Molecular Epidemiology of Mastitis Pathogens of Dairy Cattle and Comparative Relevance to Humans," *J Mammary Gland Biol Neoplasia.* 16, no. 4 (December 2011): 357–72, published online October 4, 2011.

[48] Kratz M et al., "Exchanging Carbohydrate or Protein for Fat Improves Lipid-Related Cardiovascular Risk Profile in Overweight Men and Women When Consumed *ad Libitum*," *J Investig Med.* 58, no. 5 (June 2010): 711–19.

[49] Choi HK et al., "Purine-Rich Foods, Dairy and Protein Intake, and the Risk of Gout in Men," *N Engl J Med.* 350, no. 11 (March 11, 2004): 1093–103.

[50] French SJ, Read NW. Effect of guar gum on hunger and satiety after meals of differing fat content: relationship with gastric emptying. *Am J Clin Nutr.* 1994 Jan;59(1):87–91.

[51] Ziegler EE, "Consumption of Cow's Milk as a Cause of Iron Deficiency in Infants and Toddlers," *Nutr Rev.* 69, suppl. 1 (November 2011): S37–42.

[52] Lawlor DA, Ebrahim S, Timpson N, Davey Smith G. Avoiding milk is associated with a reduced risk of insulin resistance and the metabolic syndrome: findings from the British Women's Heart and Health Study. *Diabet Med.* 2005 Jun;22(6):808–11.

[53] Bhate K, Williams HC, "Epidemiology of Acne Vulgaris," *Br J Dermatol.* (December 4, 2012), epub ahead of print.

[54] Lin SL et al., "The Role of Dairy Products and Milk in Adolescent Obesity: Evidence from Hong Kong's 'Children of 1997' Birth Cohort," *PLoS One* 7, no. 12 (2012): e52575, epub December 20, 2012.

[55] Menotti A et al., "Food Intake Patterns and 25-Year Mortality from Coronary Heart Disease: Cross-Cultural Correlations in the Seven Countries Study," The Seven Countries Study Research Group, *Eur J Epidemiol.* 15, no. 6 (July 1999): 507–15.

[56] Gu Y, Scarmeas N, "Dietary Patterns in Alzheimer's Disease and Cognitive Aging," *Curr Alzheimer Res.* 8, no. 5 (August 2011): 510–9.

[57] Paddack A et al., "Food Hypersensitivity and Otolaryngologic Conditions in Young Children," *Otolaryngol Head Neck Surg.* 147, no. 2 (August 2012): 215–20, epub March 23, 2012.

[58] Teymourpour P et al., "Cow's Milk Anaphylaxis in Children First Report of Iranian Food Allergy Registry," *Iran J Allergy Asthma Immunol.* 11, no. 1 (March 2012): 29–36.

[59] Bishop JM, Hill DJ, Hosking CS, "Natural History of Cow Milk Allergy: Clinical Outcome," *J Pediatr.* 116, no. 6 (June 1990): 862–67.

[60] Song Y et al., "Whole Milk Intake Is Associated with Prostate Cancer-Specific Mortality among US Male Physicians," *J Nutr.* 143, no. 2 (February 2013): 189–96, epub December 19, 2012.

[61] Rienks J, Dobson AJ, Mishra GD, "Mediterranean Dietary Pattern and Prevalence and Incidence of Depressive Symptoms in Mid-Aged Women: Results from a Large Community-Based Prospective Study," *Eur J Clin Nutr.* 67, no. 1 (January 2013): 75–82, epub December 5, 2012.

[62] Dean E, Gormsen Hansen R, "Prescribing Optimal Nutrition and Physical Activity as 'First-Line' Interventions for Best Practice Management of Chronic Low-Grade Inflammation Associated with Osteoarthritis: Evidence Synthesis," *Arthritis* 2012 (2012): 560634, epub December 31, 2012.

[63] Malosse D, Perron H, "Correlation Analysis between Bovine Populations, Other Farm Animals, House Pets, and Multiple Sclerosis Prevalence," *Neuroepidemiology* 12, no. 1 (1993): 15–27.

[64] Key TJ, "Diet, Insulin-Like Growth Factor-1 and Cancer Risk," *Proc Nutr Soc.* (May 3, 2011): 1–4, epub ahead of print.

[65] Chen H et al., "Consumption of Dairy Products and Risk of Parkinson's Disease," *Am J Epidemiol.* 165, no. 9 (May 1, 2007): 998–1006, epub January 31, 2007.

[66] Targher G, Byrne CD, "Nonalcoholic Fatty Liver Disease: A Novel Cardiometabolic Risk Factor for Type 2 Diabetes and Its Complications," *J Clin Endocrinol Metab.* January 4, 2013, epub ahead of print.

[67] van Faassen A et al., "The Effects of the Calcium-Restricted Diet of Urolithiasis Patients with Absorptive Hypercalciuria Type II on Risk Factors for Kidney Stones and Osteopenia," *Urol Res.* 26, no. 1 (1998): 65–69.

[68] Thiébaut AC et al., "Dietary Fatty Acids and Pancreatic Cancer in the NIH-AARP Diet and Health Study," *J Natl Cancer Inst.* 101, no. 14 (July 15, 2009): 1001–11, epub June 26, 2009.

[69] Hellgren LI, "Phytanic Acid—An Overlooked Bioactive Fatty Acid in Dairy Fat?" *Ann N Y Acad Sci.* 1190 (March 2010): 42–49.

[70] Davidson TL et al., "Intake of High-Intensity Sweeteners Alters the Ability of Sweet Taste to Signal Caloric Consequences: Implications for the Learned Control of Energy and Body Weight Regulation," *Q J Exp Psychol* (Hove) 64, no. 7 (July 2011): 1430–41.

[71] Humphries P, Pretorius E, Naudé H, "Direct and Indirect Cellular Effects of Aspartame on the Brain." *Eur J Clin Nutr.* 2008 Apr; 62(4): 451–62. Epub 2007 Aug 8.

[72] Maher TJ, Wurtman RJ, "Possible Neurologic Effects of Aspartame, a Widely Used Food Additive. "*Environ Health Perspect.* 1987 November; 75: 53–57. PMCID: PMC1474447.

[73] Schernhammer ES et al., "Consumption of Artificial Sweetener–and Sugar-Containing Soda and Risk of Lymphoma and Leukemia in Men and Women." First published October 24, 2012, doi: 10.3945/ajcn.111.030833 *Am J Clin Nutr December 2012 ajcn.030833.*

[74] Bryan GT, Yoshida O, "Artificial Sweeteners as Urinary Bladder Carcinogens." *Arch Environ Health. 1971* Jul; 23 (1): 6–12.

[75] Humphries P, Pretorius E, Naudé H, "Direct and Indirect Cellular Effects of Aspartame on the Brain." *Eur J Clin Nutr.* 2008 Apr;62(4):451–62. Epub 2007 Aug 8.

[76] Lin J, Curhan GC, "Associations of Sugar and Artificially Sweetened Soda with Albuminuria and Kidney Function Decline in Women." *Clin J Am Soc Nephrol.* 2011 January; 6(1): 160–66. doi: 10.2215/CJN.03260410. PMCID: PMC3022238.

[77] Burkhart CG, "'Lone' Atrial Fibrillation Precipitated by Monosodium Glutamate and Aspartame." *Int J Cardiol. 2009* Nov 12; 137(3): 307–8. doi: 10.1016/j.ijcard.2009.01.028. Epub 2009 Feb 10.

[78] Pretorius E, "GUT Bacteria and Aspartame: Why Are We Surprised?" *Eur J Clin Nutr.* 2012 Aug;66(8):972. doi: 10.1038/ejcn.2012.47. Epub 2012 May 16.

[79] Humphries P, Pretorius E, Naudé H, "Direct and Indirect Cellular Effects of Aspartame on the Brain." *Eur J Clin Nutr.* 2008 Apr; 62(4): 451–62. Epub 2007 Aug 8.

[80] Fengyang L, Yunhe F, Bo L, et al., "Stevioside Suppressed Inflammatory Cytokine Secretion by Downregulation of NF-κ B and MAPK Signaling Pathways in LPS-Stimulated RAW264.7 Cells," *Inflammation* 35, no. 5 (October 2012): 1669–75.

[81] Yaffe K et al., "Advanced Glycation End Product Level, Diabetes, and Accelerated Cognitive Aging," *Neurology* 77, no. 14 (October 4, 2011): 1351–56.

[82] Vlassara et al., "Protection Against Loss of Innate Defenses in Adulthood by Low Advanced Glycation End Products (AGE) Intake: Role of the Antiinflammatory AGE Receptor-1," *Journal of Clinical Endocrinology & Metabolism,* 94, no. 11 (November 2009): 4483.

[83] Lin WY et al., "Long-Term Changes in Adiposity and Glycemic Control Are Associated with Past Adenovirus Infection." *Diabetes Care.* 36, no. 3 (March 2013): 701–7.

[84] Wang C-M, Kaltenboeck B, "Exacerbation of Chronic Inflammatory Diseases by Infectious Agents: Fact or Fiction?" *World J Diabetes.* 1, no. 2 (May 15, 2010): 27–35. Published online May 15, 2010.

CHAPTER 6

[1] Rothman RB, Baumann MH, "Serotonergic Drugs and Valvular Heart Disease," *Expert Opin Drug Saf.* 8, no. 3 (May 2009): 317–29.

[2] Nihalani N et al., "Weight Gain, Obesity, and Psychotropic Prescribing," *J Obes.* (2011); 2011: 893629, published online January 17, 2011.

[3] Berman SM et al., "Potential Adverse Effects of Amphetamine Treatment on Brain and Behavior: A Review," *Mol Psychiatry.* 14, no. 2 (February 2009): 123–42, published online August 12, 2008.

[4] FDA U.S. Food and Drug Administration: http://www.accessdata.fda.gov/scripts/cdrh/cfdocs/cfCFR/CFRSearch.cfm?CFRPart=1315.

[5] Bozinovski NC et al., "The Effect of Duration of Exercise at the Ventilation Threshold on Subjective Appetite and Short-Term Food Intake in 9 to 14 Year Old Boys and Girls," *Int J Behav Nutr Phys Act.* 6 (October 9, 2009): 66, published online October 9, 2009.

[6] Kolata G, "Diabetes Study Ends Early with a Surprising Result," *New York Times Health*, October 19, 2012.

[7] From the Web site of the AANMC (Association of Accredited Naturopathic Medical Colleges), www.aanmc.org, accessed October 18, 2012, adapted.

[8] Emmerton L, Fejzic J, Tett SE, "Consumers' Experiences and Values in Conventional and Alternative Medicine Paradigms: A Problem Detection Study (PDS)," *BMC Complement Altern Med.* 12 (2012): 39, published online April 10, 2012.

[9] Burger KNJ et al., "Dietary Fiber, Carbohydrate Quality and Quantity, and Mortality Risk of Individuals with Diabetes Mellitus," *PLoS One* 7, no. 8 (2012): e43127, published online August 23, 2012.

[10] Gao X, Bermudez OI, Tucker KL. Plasma C-reactive protein and homocysteine concentrations are related to frequent fruit and vegetable intake in Hispanic and non-Hispanic white elders. *J Nutr* 2004;134:913–18.

[11] Chohan M et al., "An Investigation of the Relationship between the Anti-Inflammatory Activity, Polyphenolic Content, and Antioxidant Activities of Cooked and *In Vitro* Digested Culinary Herbs," *Oxid Med Cell Longev.* 2012 (2012): 627843, published online May 21, 2012.

[12] Janský L et al., "Immune System of Cold-Exposed and Cold-Adapted Humans," *Eur J Appl Physiol Occup Physiol.* 72, no. 5–6 (1996): 445–50.

[13] Ouellet V, Labbé SM, Blondin DP, et al. Brown adipose tissue oxidative metabolism contributes to energy expenditure during acute cold exposure in humans. *J Clin Invest.* 2012 Feb 1;122(2):545–52. doi: 10.1172/JCI60433. Epub 2012 Jan 24.

CHAPTER 7

[1] Oliveira AB et al., "The Impact of Organic Farming on Quality of Tomatoes Is Associated to Increased Oxidative Stress during Fruit Development," *PLoS One* 8, no. 2 (2013): e56354, published online February 20, 2013.

[2] Sullivan SA, Birch LL, "Infant Dietary Experience and Acceptance of Solid Foods," *Pediatrics* 93, no. 2 (February 1994): 271–77.

[3] Esposito K, Giugliano D, "Diet and Inflammation: A Link to Metabolic and Cardiovascular Diseases," *Eur Heart J.* 27, no. 1 (2006): 15–20.

[4] Lumeng CN, Saltiel AR, "Inflammatory Links between Obesity and Metabolic Disease," *J Clin Invest.* 121, no. 6 (June 1, 2011): 2111–17, published online June 1, 2011.

[5] Schulze MB et al. Dietary pattern, inflammation, and incidence of type 2 diabetes in women. *Am J Clin Nutr.* 2005 Sep;82(3):675-84; quiz 714–15.

[6] Rook GAW, "99th Dahlem Conference on Infection, Inflammation and Chronic Inflammatory Disorders: Darwinian Medicine and the 'Hygiene' or 'Old Friends' Hypothesis," *Clin Exp Immunol.* 160, no. 1 (April 2010): 70–79.

[7] Renaud S, de Lorgeril M, "Wine, Alcohol, Platelets, and the French Paradox for Coronary Heart Disease," Lancet 339, no. 8808 (June 20, 1992): 1523–26.

[8] Das DK, Mukherjee S, Ray D. "Resveratrol and Red Wine, Healthy Heart, and Longevity." *Heart Fail Rev.* 2010 Sep;15(5):467–77. doi: 10.1007/s10741-010-9163-9.

[9] Munger KL et al., "Dietary Intake of Vitamin D during Adolescence and Risk of Multiple Sclerosis," *J Neurol.* 258, no. 3 (March 2011): 479–85, published online October 14, 2010.

[10] Parikh SJ, "The Relationship between Obesity and Serum 1,25-Dihydroxy Vitamin D Concentrations in Healthy Adults," *J Clin Endocrinol Metab.* 89, no. 3 (March 2004): 1196–99.

[11] Feskanich D, Willett WC, Stampfer MJ, Colditz GA. Milk, dietary calcium, and bone fractures in women: a 12-year prospective study. *Am J Public Health* 1997;87:992–97.

[12] Martins VJB et al., "Long-Lasting Effects of Undernutrition," *Int J Environ Res Public Health* 8, no. 6 (June 2011): 1817–46, published online May 26, 2011.

[13] Ekmekcioglu C, "Are Proinflammatory Cytokines Involved in an Increased Risk for Depression by Unhealthy Diets?" *Med Hypotheses* 78, no. 2 (February 2012): 337–40, epub December 6, 2011;.

[14] de la Monte SM, "Brain Insulin Resistance and Deficiency as Therapeutic Targets in Alzheimer's Disease," *Curr Alzheimer Res.* 9, no. 1 (January 2012): 35–66, published online January 2012.

[15] Rogers AB, "Distance Burning—How Gut Microbes Promote Extraintestinal Cancers," *Gut Microbes* 2, no. 1 (January–February 2011): 52–57, published online January 1, 2011.

[16] "Stool Weights and Health," *Can Fam Physician* 22 (March 1976): 24–25.

[17] Paolini M et al., "Beta-Carotene: A Cancer Chemopreventive Agent or a Co-Carcinogen?" *Mutat Res.* 543, no. 3 (June 2003): 195–200.

[18] Spreadbury I, "Comparison with Ancestral Diets Suggests Dense Acellular Carbohydrates Promote an Inflammatory Microbiota, and May Be the Primary Dietary Cause of Leptin Resistance and Obesity," *Diabetes Metab Syndr Obes.* 5 (2012): 175–189.

[19] Santos F et al., "Functional Identification in *Lactobacillus reuteri* of a PocR-Like Transcription Factor Regulating Glycerol Utilization and Vitamin B_{12} Synthesis," *Microb Cell Fact.* 10 (2011): 55, published online July 21, 2011.

[20] Han C-c, Wei H, Guo J, "Anti-Inflammatory Effects of Fermented and Non-Fermented *Sophora flavescens*: A Comparative Study," *BMC Complement Altern Med.* 11 (2011): 100, published online October 26, 2011.

[21] Mikelsaar M, Zilmer M, "*Lactobacillus fermentum* ME-3—An Antimicrobial and Antioxidative Probiotic," *Microb Ecol Health Dis.* 21, no. 1 (April 2009): 1–27, published online March 16, 2009.

[22] Bengmark S, "Integrative Medicine and Human Health—the Role of Pre-, Pro-and Synbiotics," *Clin Transl Med.* 1 (2012): 6, published online May 28, 2012.

[23] Kwak CS et al., "Discovery of Novel Sources of Vitamin B_{12} in Traditional Korean Foods from Nutritional Surveys of Centenarians," *Curr Gerontol Geriatr Res.* 2010 (2010): 374897, published online March 8, 2011.

[24] Aggarwal J, Swami G, Kumar M, "Probiotics and Their Effects on Metabolic Diseases: An Update," *J Clin Diagn Res.* 7, no. 1 (January 2013): 173–77, published online January 1, 2013.

[25] Hodgson JM, Ward NC, Burke V, Beilin LJ, Puddey IB, "Increased Lean Red

Meat Intake Does Not Elevate Markers of Oxidative Stress and Inflammation in Humans," *J Nutr.* 137, no. 2 (2007): 363–67.

[26] Yang Q, "Gain weight by 'going diet?' Artificial sweeteners and the neurobiology of sugar cravings," *Yale J Biol Med.* 83, no. 2 (June 2010): 101–8. Published online 2010 June. PMCID: PMC2892765. *Neuroscience* 2010.

[27] Green E, Murphy C, "Altered Processing of Sweet Taste in the Brain of Diet Soda Drinkers," *Physiol Behav.* 107, no. 4 (November 5, 2012): 560–67, epub May 11, 2012.

[28] González-Castejón M, Rodriguez-Casado A, "Dietary Phytochemicals and Their Potential Effects on Obesity: A Review," *Pharmacol Res.* 64, no. 5 (November 2011): 438–55, epub Jul 21, 2011.

[29] Liu RH, "Health Benefits of Fruit and Vegetables Are from Additive and Synergistic Combinations of Phytochemicals," *Am J Clin Nutr* 78, no. 3 (September 2003): 517S–20S.

[30] Dembinska-Kiec A, Mykkänen O, Kiec-Wilk B, Mykkänen H, "Antioxidant Phytochemicals against Type 2 Diabetes," *Br J Nutr.* E Suppl. 1 (May 2008): ES109–17.

[31] Leiherer A, Mündlein A, Drexel H, "Phytochemicals and Their Impact on Adipose Tissue Inflammation and Diabetes," *Vascul Pharmacol.* 58, no. 1–2 (January 2013): 3–20, epub September 12, 2012.

[32] Janssen S et al., "Bitter Taste Receptors and α-Gustducin Regulate the Secretion of Ghrelin with Functional Effects on Food Intake and Gastric Emptying," *Proc Natl Acad Sci U S A* 108, no. 5 (February 1, 2011): 2094–99, published online January 18, 2011.

[33] Zhang C-H et al, "The Cellular and Molecular Basis of Bitter Tastant-Induced Bronchodilation." *PLoS Biol.* 2013 March; 11(3): e1001501. Published online 2013 March 5. doi: 10.1371/ journal.pbio.1001501. PMCID: PMC3589262.

[34] Li WW et al., "Tumor Angiogenesis as a Target for Dietary Cancer Prevention," *J Oncol.* 2012 (2012): 879623, published online September 29, 2011.

[35] Johnston, C, "Functional Foods as Modifiers of Cardiovascular Disease," *Am J Lifestyle Med.* 3, 1 Suppl. (July 2009): 39S–43S.

[36] Boeing H et al., "Critical Review: Vegetables and Fruit in the Prevention of Chronic Diseases," *Eur J Nutr.* 51, no. 6 (September 2012): 637–63, published online June 9, 2012.

[37] Hassan AA, Sandanger TM, Brustad M, "Level of Selected Nutrients in Meat, Liver, Tallow and Bone Marrow from Semi-Domesticated Reindeer *(Rangifer t. tarandus L.)." Int J Circumpolar Health.* 2012; 71: 10.3402/ijch.v71i0.17997. Published online 2012 March 19. doi: 10.3402/ijch.v71i0.17997. PMCID: PMC3417664.

[38] Melnik BC, "Evidence for Acne-Promoting Effects of Milk and Other Insulinotropic Dairy Products," *Nestle Nutr Workshop Ser Pediatr Program* 67 (2011): 131–45, epub Febuary 16, 2011.

[39] Herman I, *Physics of the Human Body* Springer-New York, 2007.

[40] Sparvero LJ, "Mass-Spectrometry Based Oxidative Lipidomics and Lipid Imaging: Applications in Traumatic Brain Injury," *J Neurochem.* 115, no. 6 (December 2010): 1322–36, published online November 19, 2010.

[41] Jiao L et al., "Advanced Glycation End-Products, Soluble Receptor for Advanced Glycation End-Products and Risk of Colorectal Cancer," *Cancer Epidemiol Biomarkers Prev.* 20, no. 7 (July 2011): 1430–38, published online April 28, 2011.

[42] Al-Waili NS, "Natural Honey Lowers Plasma Glucose, C-Reactive Protein,

Homocysteine, and Blood Lipids in Healthy, Diabetic, and Hyperlipidemic Subjects: Comparison with Dextrose and Sucrose," *J Med Food.* 7, no. 1 (2004): 100–7.

⁴³ http://www.diabetes.org/diabetes-basics/diabetes-myths/

⁴⁴ Dr. Duke's Phytochemical and Ethnobotanical Databases. http://sun.ars-grin. gov:8080/npgspub/xsql/duke/super2.xsql?superact=Diabetes&plants=Y&chemicals =Y&ctt=1000. Accessed April 8, 2013.

⁴⁵ Yuan G-f et al., "Effects of Different Cooking Methods on Health-Promoting Compounds of Broccoli," *J Zhejiang Univ Sci B.* 10, no. 8 (August 2009): 580–88.

CHAPTER 8

¹ Hooper PL et al., "Xenohormesis: Health Benefits from an Eon of Plant Stress Response Evolution," *Cell Stress Chaperones* 15, no. 6 (November 2010): 761–70, published online June 4, 2010.

² Bleich SN et al., "Impact of Physician BMI on Obesity Care and Beliefs," *Obesity (Silver Spring)* 20, no. 5 (May 2012): 999–1005.

³ Leiherer A, Mündlein A, Drexel H, "Phytochemicals and Their Impact on Adipose Tissue Inflammation and Diabetes," *Vascul Pharmacol.* 58, no. 1–2 (January 2013): 3–20.

⁴ CDC.gov via http://psychcentral.com/news/2011/10/25/antidepressant-use-up-400-percent-in-us/30677.html.

⁵ Schulz V, Hänsel R, Tyler VE, *Rational Phytotherapy: A Physician's Guide to Herbal Medicine.* New York, 1998.

⁶ Andallu B, Radhika B, "Hypoglycemic, Diuretic and Hypocholesterolemic Effect of Winter Cherry (*Withania somnifera, Dunal*) Root," *Indian J Exp Biol.* 38, no. 6 (June 2000): 607–9.

⁷ Williams M, "Dietary Supplements and Sports Performance: Herbals," *J Int Soc Sports Nutr.* 3, no. 1 (2006): 1–6, published online June 5, 2006.

⁸ Panossian A et al., "Adaptogens Stimulate Neuropeptide Y and Hsp72 Expression and Release in Neuroglia Cells," *Front Neurosci.* 6 (2012): 6, published online February 1, 2012, prepublished online November 12, 2011.

⁹ Hofseth LJ, "Nitric Oxide as a Target of Complementary and Alternative Medicines to Prevent and Treat Inflammation and Cancer," *Cancer Lett.* 268, no. 1 (September 8, 2008): 10–30, published online April 25, 2008.

¹⁰ Jia L, Zhao Y, Liang X-J, "Current Evaluation of the Millennium Phytomedicine—Ginseng (II): Collected Chemical Entities, Modern Pharmacology, and Clinical Applications Emanated from Traditional Chinese Medicine," *Curr Med Chem.* 16, no. 22 (2009): 2924–42.

¹¹ Wu Z, Luo JZ, Luo L, "American Ginseng Modulates Pancreatic Beta Cell Activities," *Chin Med.* 2 (2007): 11, published online October 25, 2007.

¹² Huyen VTT et al., "Antidiabetic Effects of Add-On *Gynostemma pentaphyllum* Extract Therapy with Sulfonylureas in Type 2 Diabetic Patients," *Evid Based Complement Alternat Med.* 2012 (2012): 452313, published online October 17, 2012.

¹³ Weidner C et al., "Amorfrutins are Potent Antidiabetic Dietary Natural Products," *Proc Natl Acad Sci U S A.* 109, no. 19 (May 8, 2012): 7257–7262, published online April 16, 2012.

[14] Su CH, Lai MN, Ng LT, "Inhibitory Effects of Medicinal Mushrooms on α-Amylase and α-Glucosidase - Enzymes Related to Hyperglycemia," *Food Funct.* February 8, 2013, epub ahead of print.

[15] Yarnell E, Abascal K, Hooper CG, *Clinical Botanical Medicine.* Larchmont NY, Mary Anne Liebert, Inc. publishers: 2003.

[16] Perera PK, Yunman Li Y, "Functional Herbal Food Ingredients Used in Type 2 Diabetes Mellitus," *Pharmacogn Rev.* 6, no. 11 (January–June 2012): 37–45.

[17] Winston D, Maines S, *Adaptogens: Herbs for Strength, Stamina and Stress Relief.* Rochester VT, Healing Arts Press: 2007.

[18] Ohsugi M, Fan W, Hase K, Xiong Q, Tezuka Y, Komatsu K, et al., "Active Oxygen Scavenging Activity of Traditional Nourishing-Tonic Herbal Medicines and Active Constituents of Rhodiola Sacra," *J Ethnopharmacology* 67 (1999): 111–19.

[19] Duke JA, *The Green Pharmacy: The Ultimate Compendium of Natural Remedies from the World's Foremost Authority on Healing Herbs.* New York, St. Martin's Paperbacks: 1998.

[20] Jo S-H et al., "*In Vitro* and *in Vivo* Anti-Hyperglycemic Effects of Omija (*Schizandra chinensis*) Fruit," *Int J Mol Sci.* 12, no. 2 (2011): 1359–70, published online February 23, 2011.

[21] Wang R et al., "A Survey of Chinese Herbal Ingredients with Liver Protection Activities," *Chin Med.* 2 (2007): 5, published online May 10, 2007.

[22] Duke JA, *The Green Pharmacy: The Ultimate Compendium of Natural Remedies from the World's Foremost Authority on Healing Herbs.* New York, 1998.

[23] Bäumler S, *Heilpflanzen Praxis Heute: Porträts—Rezepturen—Anwendung.* München, Elsevier: 2007, 701.

[24] Blumenthal M et al. (ed), *The Complete German Commision E Monographs. Therapeutic Guide to Herbal Medicines.* Austin TX, Thieme Medical Publishers Inc.: 1998.

[25] Namazi N, Esfanjani AT, Heshmati J, Bahrami A, "The Effect of Hydro Alcoholic Nettle (*Urtica dioica*) Extracts on Insulin Sensitivity and Some Inflammatory Indicators in Patients with Type 2 Diabetes: A Randomized Double-Blind Control Trial," *Pak J Biol Sci.* 14, no. 15 (August 1, 2011): 775–79.

[26] Ozkarsli M, Sevim H, Sen A, "In Vivo Effects of *Urtica urens* (Dwarf Nettle) on the Expression of CYP1A in Control and 3-Methylcholanthrene-Exposed Rats," *Xenobiotica* 38, no. 1 (January 2008): 48–61.

[27] Watanabe T et al., "Effects of Oral Administration of *Pfaffia paniculata* (Brazilian Ginseng) on Incidence of Spontaneous Leukemia in AKR/J Mice," *Cancer Detect Prev.* 24, no. 2 (2000): 173–78.

[28] Kim I-S et al., "Antioxidant Activities of Hot Water Extracts from Various Spices," *Int J Mol Sci.* 12, no. 6 (2011): 4120–31, published online June 21, 2011.

[29] El-Beshbishy H, Bahashwan S, "Hypoglycemic Effect of Basil (*Ocimum basilicum*) Aqueous Extract Is Mediated through Inhibition of α-glucosidase and α-Amylase Activities: An in Vitro Study," *Toxicol Ind Health.* 28, no. 1 (February 2012): 42–50, epub June 2, 2011.

[30] Benzie IFF (ed), Wachtel-Galor S (ed), *Herbal Medicine: Biomolecular and Clinical Aspects.* 2nd edition. Boca Raton: CRC Press; 2011, chapter 4.

[31] Kolehmainen M, Mykkänen O, Kirjavainen PV et al., "Bilberries Reduce Low-Grade Inflammation in Individuals with Features of Metabolic Syndrome," *Mol Nutr Food Res.* 56, no. 10 (October 2012): 1501–10, epub September 7, 2012.

[32] Helmstädter A, Schuster N, "*Vaccinium myrtillus* as an Antidiabetic Medicinal Plant—Research through the Ages," *Pharmazie.* 65, no. 5 (May 2010): 315–21.

[33] Srivastava Y, "Antidiabetic and Adaptogenic Properties of *Momordica charantia* Extract: An Experimental and Clinical Evaluation," *Phytother Res.* 7 (1993): 285–89.

[34] Chaturvedi P, "Antidiabetic Potentials of *Momordica charantia*: Multiple Mechanisms behind the Effects," *J Med Food.* 15, no. 2 (February 2012): 101–7.

[35] Aggarwal BB et al., "Identification of Novel Anti-Inflammatory Agents from Ayurvedic Medicine for Prevention of Chronic Diseases," *Curr Drug Targets.* 12, no. 11 (October 1, 2011): 1595–1653.

[36] Park U-H et al., "Piperine, a Component of Black Pepper, Inhibits Adipogenesis by Antagonizing PPARγ Activity in 3T3-L1 Cells," *J. Agric. Food Chem.* 60, no. 15 (2012): 3853–60.

[37] Chan YS et al., "A Review of the Pharmacological Effects of *Arctium lappa* (Burdock)," *Inflammopharmacology* 19, no. 5 (October 2011): 245–54, epub October 28, 2010.

[38] Johri RK, "*Cuminum cyminum* and *Carum carvi*: An Update," *Pharmacogn Rev.* 5, no. 9 (January–June 2011): 63–72.

[39] Vasanthi HR, Parameswari RP, "Indian Spices for Healthy Heart—An Overview," *Curr Cardiol Rev.* 6, no. 4 (November 2010): 274–79.

[40] Chaiyata P, Puttadechakum S, Komindr S, "Effect of Chili Pepper (*Capsicum frutescens*) Ingestion on Plasma Glucose Response and Metabolic Rate in Thai Women," *J Med Assoc Thai.* 86, no. 9 (September 2003): 854–60.

[41] Srivastava JK, Shankar E, Gupta S, "Chamomile: A Herbal Medicine of the Past with Bright Future," *Mol Med Report.* 3, no. 6 (November 1, 2010): 895–901.

[42] Adamsson V et al., "What Is a Healthy Nordic Diet? Foods and Nutrients in the NORDIET Study," *Food Nutr Res.* 56 (2012), published online June 27, 2012.

[43] Kowalchik C (ed), Hylton WH (ed), *Rodale's Illustrated Encyclopedia of Herbs.* Emmaus, PA: Rodale, 1987.

[44] Leach MJ, Kumar S, "Cinnamon for Diabetes Mellitus," *Cochrane Database Syst Rev.* 9 (2012).

[45] Akilen R et al., "Cinnamon in Glycaemic Control: Systematic Review and Meta Analysis," *Clin Nutr.* 31, no. 5 (2012): 609–15.

[46] Jagtap AG, Patil PB, "Antihyperglycemic Activity and Inhibition of Advanced Glycation End Product Formation by *Cuminum cyminum* in Streptozotocin Induced Diabetic Rats," *Food Chem Toxicol.* 48, no. 8–9 (August–September 2010), epub May 6, 2010.

[47] Dhandapani S et al., "Hypolipidemic Effect of *Cuminum cyminum* L. on Alloxan-Induced Diabetic Rats," *Pharmacol Res.* 46, no. 3 (September 2002): 251–55.

[48] Scalzo R, Cronin M, *Herbal Solutions for Healthy Living. A Practical Guide to Using Herbal Solutions Safely and Effectively.* Brevard, NC: Herbal Research Publications, 2001.

[49] Zhang J et al., "Pancreatic Lipase Inhibitory Activity of *Taraxacum officinale in Vitro* and *in Vivo*," *Nutr Res Pract.* 2, no. 4 (Winter 2008): 200–3, published online December 31, 2008.

[50] Birkhan H, *Pflanzen im Mittelalter—Eine Kulturgeschichte*. Wien–Köln–Weimar, Böhlau Verlag Wien, 2012.

[51] Panda S, "The Effect of *Anethum graveolens L.* (Dill) on Corticosteroid Induced Diabetes Mellitus: Involvement of Thyroid Hormones," *Phytother Res.* 22, no. 12 (December 2008): 1695–97.

[52] http://www.ars-grin.gov/duke/

[53] Kunzemann J, Herrmann K, "Isolation and Identification of Flavon(ol)-Glycosides in Caraway (*Carum carvi* L.), Fennel (*Foeniculum vulgare* Mill.), Anise (*Pimpinella anisum* L.), and Coriander (*Coriandrum sativum* L.), and of Flavon-c-glycosides in Anise I Phenolics of Spices," *A. Lebensm Unters Forsch.* 164 (1977): 194–200.

[54] Aggarwal BB et al., "Identification of Novel Anti-Inflammatory Agents from Ayurvedic Medicine for Prevention of Chronic Diseases," *Curr Drug Targets.* 12, no. 11 (October 1, 2011): 1595–1653.

[55] Gupta A, Gupta R, Lal B, "Effect of *Trigonella foenum-graecum* (Fenugreek) Seeds on Glycaemic Control and Insulin Resistance in Type 2 Diabetes Mellitus: A Double Blind Placebo Controlled Study," *J Assoc Physicians India.* 49 (November 2001): 1057–61.

[56] Kaefer CM, Milner JA, "The Role of Herbs and Spices in Cancer Prevention," *J Nutr Biochem.* 19, no. 6 (June 2008): 347–61.

[57] Aggarwal BB et al., "Identification of Novel Anti-Inflammatory Agents from Ayurvedic Medicine for Prevention of Chronic Diseases," *Curr Drug Targets.* 12, no. 11 (October 1, 2011): 1595–1653.

[58] Kumar R et al., "Antihyperglycemic, Antihyperlipidemic, Anti-Inflammatory and Adenosine Deaminase-Lowering Effects of Garlic in Patients with Type 2 Diabetes Mellitus with Obesity," *Diabetes Metab Syndr Obes.* 6 (2013): 49–56, epub January 19, 2013.

[59] Kaefer CM, Milner JA, "The Role of Herbs and Spices in Cancer Prevention," *J Nutr Biochem.* 19, no. 6 (June 2008): 347–61.

[60] Li Y et al., "Preventive and Protective Properties of *Zingiber officinale* (Ginger) in Diabetes Mellitus, Diabetic Complications, and Associated Lipid and Other Metabolic Disorders: A Brief Review," *Evid Based Complement Alternat Med.* 2012 (2012): 516870, published online November 22, 2012.

[61] Mansour MS et al. Ginger consumption enhances the thermic effect of food and promotes feelings of satiety without affecting metabolic and hormonal parameters in overweight men: A pilot study. *Metabolism.* 2012, doi:10.1016/j.metabol.2012.03.016.

[62] Andallu B, Radhika B, and Suryakantham V, "Effect of aswagandha, ginger and mulberry on hyperglycemia and hyperlipidemia," *Plant Foods for Human Nutrition*, vol. 58, no. 3, pp. 1–7, 2003.

[63] Megha Saraswat M et al., "Antiglycating Potential of *Zingiber officinalis* and Delay of Diabetic Cataract in Rats," *Mol Vis.* 16 (2010): 1525–37, published online August 10, 2010.

[64] Birks J, Grimley EV, Van Dongen M, "Ginkgo Biloba for Cognitive Impairment and Dementia," *Cochrane Database Syst Rev.* 2002: CD003120.

[65] Muir AH, Robb R, McLaren M et al., "The Use of *Ginkgo biloba* in Raynaud's Disease: A Double-Blind Placebo-Controlled Trial," *Vasc Med.* 7, no. 4 (2002): 265–67.

[66] Kanetkar P, Singhal R, Kamat M, "*Gymnema sylvestre*: A Memoir," *J Clin Biochem Nutr.* 41, no. 2 (September 2007): 77–81, published online August 29, 2007.

[67] Sharafi SM et al., "Protective Effects of Bioactive Phytochemicals from *Mentha piperita* with Multiple Health Potentials," *Pharmacogn Mag.* 6, no. 23 (July–September 2010): 147–53.

[68] Hanhineva K et al., "Impact of Dietary Polyphenols on Carbohydrate Metabolism," *Int J Mol Sci.* 11, no. 4 (2010): 1365–1402, published online March 31, 2010.

[69] Johnson JJ, "Carnosol: A promising Anti-Cancer and Anti-Inflammatory Agent," *Cancer Lett.* 305, no. 1 (June 1, 2011): 1–7, published online March 5, 2011.

[70] Sá CM et al., "Sage Tea Drinking Improves Lipid Profile and Antioxidant Defences in Humans," *Int J Mol Sci.* 10, no 9 (September 2009): 3937–50, published online September 9, 2009.

[71] Maryam Shekarchi M et al., "Comparative Study of Rosmarinic Acid Content in Some Plants of Labiatae Family," *Pharmacogn Mag.* 8, no. 29 (January–March 2012): 37–41.

[72] Eckert GP, "Traditional Used Plants against Cognitive Decline and Alzheimer Disease," *Front Pharmacol.* 1 (2010): 138, published online December 8, 2010.

[73] Maryam Shekarchi M et al., "Comparative Study of Rosmarinic Acid Content in Some Plants of Labiatae Family," *Pharmacogn Mag.* 8, no. 29 (January–March 2012): 37–41.

[74] Anton SD et al., "Effects of Stevia, Aspartame, and Sucrose on Food Intake, Satiety, and Postprandial Glucose and Insulin Levels," *Appetite.* 55, no. 1 (August 2010): 37–43, published online March 18, 2010.

[75] Eisenman SW et al., "Qualitative Variation of Anti-Diabetic Compounds in Different Tarragon (*Artemisia dracunculus* L.) Cytotypes," *Fitoterapia.* 82, no. 7 (October 2011): 1062–74, published online July 21, 2011.

[76] Ocaña A, Reglero G, "Effects of Thyme Extract Oils (from *Thymus vulgaris, Thymus zygis,* and *Thymus hyemalis*) on Cytokine Production and Gene Expression of oxLDL-Stimulated THP-1-Macrophages," *J Obes.* 2012 (2012): 104706, published online April 17, 2012.

[77] Shehzad A, Rehman G, Lee YS, "Curcumin in Inflammatory Diseases," *Biofactors* 39, no. 1 (January 2013): 69–77, epub December 22, 2012.

[78] Sahebkar A, "Why It Is Necessary to Translate Curcumin into Clinical Practice for the Prevention and Treatment of Metabolic Syndrome?" *Biofactors* December 13, 2012.

[79] Chuengsamarn S, Rattanamongkolgul S, Luechapudiporn R, Phisalaphong C, Jirawatnotai S. Curcumin Extract for Prevention of Type 2 Diabetes. *Diabetes Care.* 2012 Jul 6.

[80] Guo AJ et al., "Stimulation of Apolipoprotein A-IV Expression in Caco-2/TC7 Enterocytes and Reduction of Triglyceride Formation in 3T3-L1 Adipocytes by Potential Anti-Obesity Chinese Herbal Medicines," *Chin Med.* 4 (2009): 5, published online March 26, 2009.

CHAPTER 9

[1] Metcalfe RS et al., "Towards the Minimal Amount of Exercise for Improving Metabolic Health: Beneficial Effects of Reduced-Exertion High-Intensity Interval Training," *Eur J Appl Physiol.* 112, no. 7 (July 2012): 2767–75, epub November 29, 2011.

[2] O'Keefe JH et al., "Potential Adverse Cardiovascular Effects from Excessive Endurance Exercise," *Mayo Clin Proc.* 87, no. 6 (June 2012): 587–95.

[3] Ford ES, "Does Exercise Reduce Inflammation? Physical Activity and C-Reactive Protein among U.S. Adults," *Epidemiology* 13, no. 5 (September 2002).

[4] Teixeira-Lemos E et al., "Regular Physical Exercise Training Assists in Preventing Type 2 Diabetes Development: Focus on Its Antioxidant and Anti-Inflammatory Properties," *Cardiovasc Diabetol.* 10 (2011): 12, published online January 28, 2011.

[5] Fisher-Wellman K, Bloomer RJ, "Acute Exercise and Oxidative Stress: A 30 Year History," *Dyn Med.* 8 (2009): 1, published online January 13, 2009.

[6] Tapia PC, "Sublethal Mitochondrial Stress with an Attendant Stoichiometric Augmentation of Reactive Oxygen Species May Precipitate Many of the Beneficial Alterations in Cellular Physiology Produced by Caloric Restriction, Intermittent Fasting, Exercise and Dietary Phytonutrients: 'Mitohormesis' for Health and Vitality," *Medical Hypotheses* 66, no. 4 (2006): 832–43.

[7] Perls T, Terry D, "Understanding the Determinants of Exceptional Longevity," *Ann Intern Med.* 139, no. 5, part 2 (September 2, 2003): 445–49.

[8] Thompson Coon J, "Does Participating in Physical Activity in Outdoor Natural Environments Have a Greater Effect on Physical and Mental Wellbeing Than Physical Activity Indoors? A Systematic Review," *Environ Sci Technol.* 45, no. 5 (March 1, 2011): 1761–72, epub February 3, 2011.

[9] Cider Å et al., "Aquatic Exercise Is Effective in Improving Exercise Performance in Patients with Heart Failure and Type 2 Diabetes Mellitus," *Evid Based Complement Alternat Med.* 2012; 2012: 349209, published online April 23, 2012.

[10] Erickson KI et al., "Physical Activity Predicts Gray Matter Volume in Late Adulthood. The Cardiovascular Health Study," *Neurology* 75, no. 16 (October 19, 2010): 1415–22.

[11] Morrison K et al., "Effect of a Sand or Firm-Surface Walking Program on Health, Strength, and Fitness in Women 60–75 Years Old," *J Aging Phys Act.* 17, no. 2 (April 2009): 196–209.

[12] Bankoski A et al., "Sedentary Activity Associated With Metabolic Syndrome Independent of Physical Activity," *Diabetes Care.* 34, no. 2 (February 2011): 497–503, published online January 20, 2011.

[13] Helmerhorst HJ, Wijndaele K, Brage S, Wareham NJ, Ekelund U. Objectively measured sedentary time may predict insulin resistance independent of moderate- and vigorous-intensity physical activity. *Diabetes* 2009;58:1776–79.

[14] Flanagan S et al., "Squatting Exercises in Older Adults: Kinematic and Kinetic Comparisons," *Med Sci Sports Exerc.* 35, no. 4 (April 2003): 635–43.

[15] de Brito LB et al., "Ability to Sit and Rise from the Floor as a Predictor of All-Cause Mortality," *Eur J Prev Cardiol.* December 13, 2012, epub ahead of print.

[16] Black DS, Cole SW, Irwin MR, et al., "Yogic Meditation Reverses NFκ B and IRF-Related Transcriptome Dynamics in Leukocytes of Family Dementia Caregivers

in a Randomized Controlled Trial," *Psychoneuroendocrinology* 38, no. 3 (March 2013): 348–55.

CHAPTER 10

[1] Gagnon C, Lu ZX, Magliano DJ, et al., "Low Serum 25-hydroxyvitamin D Is Associated with Increased Risk of the Development of the Metabolic Syndrome at Five Years: Results from a National, Population-Based Prospective Study." [The Australian Diabetes, Obesity, and Lifestyle Study: AusDiab.] *J Clin Endocrinol Metab*, 97, no. 6 (June 2012): 1953–61.

[2] Belenchia AM, Tosh AK, Hillman LS, Peterson CA, "Correcting Vitamin D Insufficiency Improves Insulin Sensitivity in Obese Adolescents: A Randomized Controlled Trial," *Am J Clin Nutr.* (February 13, 2013), epub ahead of print.

[3] Satish U et al., "Is CO2 an Indoor Pollutant? Direct Effects of Low-to-Moderate CO2 Concentrations on Human Decision-Making Performance," *Environ Health Perspect.* September 20, 2012, epub ahead of print, October 28, 2012.

[4] Kiecolt-Glaser JK, Preacher KJ, MacCallum RC, Atkinson C, Malarkey WB, Glaser R, "Chronic Stress and Age-Related Increases in the Proinflammatory Cytokine Interleukin-6," *Proceedings of the National Academy of Sciences, USA* 100, no. 15 (July 22, 2003): 9090–95.

CHAPTER 11

[1] Hue O et al., "The Effect of Time-of-Day on Cold Water Ingestion by High-Level Swimmers in Tropical Climate," *Int J Sports Physiol Perform*, January 4, 2013, epub ahead of print.

[2] Kaptchuk T, *The Web That Has No Weaver: Understanding Chinese Medicine* New York: McGraw-Hill, 1983), NEED PAGE NUMBERS.

[3] Bougault V, Boulet LP, "Airway Dysfunction in Swimmers," *Br J Sports Med.* 46, no. 6 (May 2012): 402–6, epub January 12, 2012.

[4] Zhao Y et al., "Occurrence and Formation of Chloro- and Bromo-Benzoquinones during Drinking Water Disinfection," *Water Res.* 46, no. 14 (September 15, 2012): 4351–60, epub June 2, 2012.

[5] Lord K et al., "Environmentally Persistent Free Radicals Decrease Cardiac Function before and after Ischemia/Reperfusion Injury in Vivo," *J Recept Signal Transduct Res.* 31, no. 2 (April 2011): 157–67.

[6] Reis MA et al., "High Airborne PM2.5 Chlorine Concentrations Link to Diabetes Surge in Portugal," *Sci Total Environ.* 407, no. 21 (October 15, 2009): 5726–34, epub August 15, 2009.

[7] Lablanche S et al., "Protection of Pancreatic INS-1 β-cells from Glucose- and Fructose-Induced Cell Death by Inhibiting Mitochondrial Permeability Transition with Cyclosporin A or Metformin," *Cell Death Dis.* 2, no. 3 (March 2011): e134, published online March 24, 2011.

[8] Higdon JV, Frei B., "Coffee and Health: A Review of Recent Human Research," *Crit Rev Food Sci Nutr.* 46, no. 2 (2006): 101–23.

[9] Pimentel GD et al., "Does Long-Term Coffee Intake Reduce Type 2 Diabetes Mellitus Risk?" *Diabetology & Metabolic Syndrome* 1 (2009): 6.

[10] Chu YF et al., "Roasted Coffees High in Lipophilic Antioxidants and Chlorogenic Acid Lactones Are More Neuroprotective Than Green Coffees," *J Agric Food Chem.* 57, no. 20 (October 28, 2009): 9801–8.

[11] Laestadius JG, Dimberg L, "Hot Water for Handwashing—Where Is the Proof?," *J Occup Environ Med.* 47, no. 4 (April 2005): 434–35.

[12] Rayfield EJ et al., "Infection and Diabetes: The Case for Glucose Control," *Am J Med.* 72, no. 3 (March 1982): 439–50.

[13] Lee P et al., "Mild Cold Exposure Modulates Fibroblast Growth Factor 21 (FGF21) Diurnal Rhythm in Humans: Relationship between FGF21 Levels, Lipolysis, and Cold-Induced Thermogenesis," *J Clin Endocrinol Metab.* 98, no. 1 (January 2013): E98–102, epub November 12, 2012.

[14] Castellani JW et al., "Human Thermoregulatory Responses during Serial Cold-Water Immersions," *Journal of Applied Physiology* 85, no. 1 (July 1, 1998): 204-9.

[15] Fleckenstein A, Weisman R, Health$_2$O—Tap into the Healing Powers of Water. 2007.

[16] Thormar H (ed), *Lipids and Essential Oils as Antimicrobial Agents* (New York: Wiley, 2011).

[17] Koraλ RR, Khambholja KM, "Potential of Herbs in Skin Protection from Ultraviolet Radiation," *Pharmacogn Rev.* 5, no. 10 (July–December 2011): 164–73.

CHAPTER 12

[1] Dori E, Rosenberg DE et al., "Brief Scales to Assess Physical Activity and Sedentary Equipment in the Home," *Int J Behav Nutr Phys Act.* 7 (2010): 10, published online January 31, 2010.

APPENDIX

[1] Obrenovich ME et al., "Antioxidants in Health, Disease, and Aging," *CNS Neurol Disord Drug Targets* 10, no. 2 (March 2011): 192–207.

[2] Koltai E et al., "Age-Associated Declines in Mitochondrial Biogenesis and Protein Quality Control Factors Are Minimized by Exercise Training," *Am J Physiol Regul Integr Comp Physiol.* 303, no. 2 (July 15, 2012): R127-34, epub May 9, 2012.

[3] Yin D, "Is Carbonyl Detoxification an Important Anti-Aging Process during Sleep?" *Med Hypotheses* 54, no. 4 (April 2000): 519–22.

[4] Khan N, Mukhtar H, "Tea and Health: Studies in Humans," *Curr Pharm Des.* February 19, 2013, epub ahead of print.

[5] Mattson MP, "Does Brown Fat Protect Against Diseases of Aging?" *Ageing Res Rev.* 9, no. 1 (January 2010): 69, published online December 5, 2009.

[6] Kyriazis M, "Clinical Anti-Aging Hormetic Strategies," *Rejuvenation Res.* 8, no. 2 (Summer 2005): 96–100.

[7] Pan MH et al., "Molecular Mechanisms for Anti-Aging by Natural Dietary Compounds," *Mol Nutr Food Res.* 56, no. 1 (January 2012): 88–115, epub November 14, 2011.

[8] Lima CF, Pereira-Wilson C, Rattan SI, "Curcumin Induces Heme Oxygenase-1 in Normal Human Skin Fibroblasts through Redox Signaling: Relevance for Anti-Aging Intervention," *Mol Nutr Food Res.* 55, no. 3 (March 2011): 430–42, epub October 11, 2010.

[9] Cotman CW, Berchtold NC, Christie LA, "Exercise Builds Brain Health: Key Roles of Growth Factor Cascades and Inflammation," *Trends Neurosci.* 30, no. 9 (September 2007): 464–72, epub August 31, 2007.

[10] Lue L-F et al., "Is There Inflammatory Synergy in Type II Diabetes Mellitus and Alzheimer's Disease?" *Int J Alzheimers Dis.* 2012 (2012): 918680, published online June 21, 2012.

[11] Knott L et al., "Regulation of Osteoarthritis by Omega-3 (n-3) Polyunsaturated Fatty Acids in a Naturally Occurring Model of Disease," *Osteoarthritis and Cartilage*, 19, no. 9, September 2011.

[12] Duval C et al., "The Effect of Trager Therapy on the Level of Evoked Stretch Responses in Patients with Parkinson's Disease and Rigidity," *J Manipulative Physiol Ther.* 25, no. 7 (September 2002): 455–64.

[13] Forst T et al., "Pilot Study for the Evaluation of Morphological and Functional Changes in Retinal Blood Flow in Patients with Insulin Resistance and/or Type 2 Diabetes Mellitus," *J Diabetes Sci Technol.* 6, no. 1 (January 2012): 163–68, published online January 1, 2012.

[14] Foos RY et al., "Posterior Vitreous Detachment in Diabetic Subjects," *Ophthalmology* 87, no. 2 (February 1980): 122–28.

[15] Yang Y et al., "Retinal Redox Stress and Remodeling in Cardiometabolic Syndrome and Diabetes," *Oxid Med Cell Longev.* 3, no. 6 (November–December 2010): 392–403.

[16] Choudhury F et al., "Risk Factors for Four-Year Incidence and Progression of Age-Related Macular Degeneration: The Los Angeles Latino Eye Study," *Am J Ophthalmol.* 152, no. 3 (September 2011): 385–95, published online June 16, 2011.

[17] Richter GM et al., "Risk Factors for Cortical, Nuclear, Posterior Subcapsular, and Mixed Lens Opacities: The Los Angeles Latino Eye Study," *Ophthalmology* 119, no. 3 (March 2012): 547–54, published online December 23, 2011.

[18] Newman-Casey PA, "The Relationship between Components of Metabolic Syndrome and Open-Angle Glaucoma," *Ophthalmology* 118, no. 7 (July 2011): 1318–26, published online April 9, 2011.

[19] Chen H et al., "A Microalbuminuria Threshold to Predict the Risk for the Development of Diabetic Retinopathy in Type 2 Diabetes Mellitus Patients," *PLoS One* 7, no. 5 (2012): e36718, published online May 10, 2012.

[20] Siegel R, Naishadham D, Jemal A, "Cancer Statistics, 2012," *CA Cancer J Clin.* 62, no. 1 (January–February 2012): 10–29, epub January 4, 2012.

[21] http://www.win.niddk.nih.gov/statistics/, accessed April 24, 2013.

[22] Park HK, "Metformin and Cancer in Type 2 Diabetes." *Diabetes Metab J.* 2013 April; 37(2): 113–16. Published online 2013 April 16. doi: 10.4093/dmj.2013.37.2.113. PMCID: PMC3638221.

[23] Hemminki K et al., "Risk of Cancer Following Hospitalization for Type 2 Diabetes," *The Oncologist* 15, no. 6 (June 2010): 548–55.

[24] Graham NA et al., "Glucose Deprivation Activates a Metabolic and Signaling Amplification Loop Leading to Cell Death," *Mol Syst Biol.* 8 (June 26, 2012): 589.

[25] Centers for Disease and Prevention. "Vaccine Effectiveness—How Well the Flu Vaccine Works? Questions and Answers." Accessed June 11, 2003. http://www.cdc.gov/flu/about/qa/vaccineeffect.htm#howeffectiveelderly

[26] J. Rafferty J, Tsikoudas A, Davis BC, "Ear Candling—Should General Practitioners Recommend It?" *Can Fam Physician* 53, no. 12 (December 2007): 2121–22.

[27] Iabichella ML, "The Use of an Extract of *Hypericum perforatum* and *Azadirachta indica* in Advanced Diabetic Foot: An Unexpected Outcome," *BMJ Case Rep.* (February 2013): 2013.

[28] Charoenkiatkul S et al., "Calcium Absorption from Commonly Consumed Vegetables in Healthy Thai Women," *J Food Sci.* 73, no. 9 (November 2008): H218-21.

[29] Haron H et al., "Absorption of Calcium from Milk and Tempeh Consumed by Postmenopausal Malay Women Using the Dual Stable Isotope Technique," *Int J Food Sci Nutr.* 61, no. 2 (March 2010): 125–37.

[30] David A Rosen DA et al, "Detection of Intracellular Bacterial Communities in Human Urinary Tract Infection." *PLoS Med.* 2007 December; 4(12): e329. Published online 2007 December 18. doi: 10.1371/ journal.pmed.0040329. PMCID: PMC2140087.

[31] Head KA, "Natural Approaches to Prevention and Treatment of Infections of the Lower Urinary Tract," *Altern Med Rev.* 13, no. 3 (September 2008): 227–44.

INDEX

<u>Underscored</u> page references indicate boxed text. **Boldface** references indicate illustrations.

A

Abalone, 103
Abdominal discomfort/pain, <u>46</u>, <u>127</u>, <u>297</u>
Abdominal strength, exercise for, 145
Abuse, 45–46
Acanthosis nigricans, <u>5</u>
Acellular foods, 87
Acne, <u>296</u>
Actos, 30
Acute conditions, 74, <u>75</u>, 138
ADA (American Diabetes Association), 110–111
Adaptogens, 122–123
Addictive foods, grains as, 64
Adenosine-5-triphosphate (ATP), <u>34</u>
Adipokines, 55, 56–57
Adult-onset diabetes. *See* Diabetes, Type 2
Advanced glycation end products (AGEs), 66, 107, 132
Advertising, 39–40
Aerobic respiration, <u>34</u>, 35
Age, as diabetes risk factor, <u>4</u>
AGEs (advanced glycation end products), 66, 107, 132
Aging, premature, 271–273
Agricultural subsidies, 39–40
Alcohol, 83, 94, 167–168
Allergies. *See* Food allergies
Aloe vera, 293, 298–299
Alpha-glucosidase inhibitors, 30
Alternative medicine, 120
Alzheimer's disease, 273
Amaranth, <u>236</u>
American Diabetes Association (ADA), 110–11
Anethole, 131
Animal fat, 62–63, 91
Anthocyanins, <u>51</u>, 128
Anti-aging, herbs/spices for, 272–273
Antibiotics, 293

Anticoagulants, 297
Antidepressants, 121
Anti-diabetic medications, 28–31
Anti-inflammatory diet
  benefits, 83
  case histories, <u>95</u>
  customization of, 80
  foods in, 89–91
  phytonutrients in, 87
  supplements for, 274
  Weekend Jump Start plan, 182–188
Antinutrients, 63–64, 89, 90
Antioxidants, <u>9</u>, <u>51</u>, 168
Antiseptics, plant-based, <u>296</u>, <u>299</u>
A1c, <u>16–17</u>, 22
Appetite suppressants, 72. *See also* Hunger
Apples
  Baked Apples, 262
  Crustless Apple Pie, 263
  Fruit Smoothie, 264
  shopping/storage tips, <u>255</u>
Apricots, <u>255</u>
Arm extensions exercise, 149
Aromatherapy, <u>297</u>
Arterial disease, 273–274
Arthritis, <u>93</u>, <u>157</u>, <u>169</u>, 274
Artichokes, <u>218</u>
Artificial sweeteners, 65–66, 92, 168
Arugula
  Easy Arugula Salad with Egg, <u>216</u>
  preparation suggestions, <u>214</u>
Ashwaganda, 124
Asparagus, <u>218</u>
Asthma, 65
Astragalus, 124
Astronaut food, 86
Athlete's foot, 274–275
ATP (adenosine-5-triphosphate), <u>34</u>
Atrazine, 61–62
Attentiveness, to eating, 183
Autonomic nervous system, 59

F

Fall risks, reducing, 148
Family history
    as diabetes risk factor, 4, 7
    eating habits, 42–43, 45–46
Family meals, 113
Farro, 236
Fasting
    after dinner/overnight, 43, 113–114, 114
    for toxin elimination, 59
Fasting blood sugar test, 16
Fatigue
    diabetes-caused, 32
    eliminating, 35–38
    hunger role, 43–44
    metabolism and, 33–35
    as sign of food allergy, 46
    tonics for, 124, 125
Fatty liver, 168
Fennel, 130–131, 132, 220
Fenugreek, 131
Fermented foods, 90, 105
FGF21 protein, 171–172
Fight-or-flight response, 59
Figs, 256
Fish and seafood
    cooking guidelines, 251
    farm-raised, as pro-inflammatory food, 94
    recipes
        Broiled Trout, 252
        Cod and Shrimp Stew, 252
        Grilled Miso-Glazed Salmon, 253
        Sautéed Monkfish Fillets, 253
        Shrimp Salad, 254
    sourcing/shopping tips, 91, 94, 102, 103, 116
Fish oils, 278, 287, 300
Fitness, in midlife, 21. See also Exercise
Five Health Essentials
    balance, 156–163
    food, 79–88
    herbs and spices, 119–135
    overview, 76–77, 155
    water, 165–177
    in Weekend Jump Start, 184
Five Tibetan Rites, 143–146, 200
Flavonoids, 51, 97
Flexible eating. See Rotation, of foods

Flu, 282–283
Fluid intake, 39. See also Water, drinking of
Food
    availability, 35, 44
    color of, 50, 51
    cost of, 116–117
    freshness, 83–88, 113
    as Health Essential, 77–78
    healthy vs. unhealthy, 80
    meal planning guidelines, 80–81
    as source of body fat, 21
    texture of, 50
    in two week sample plan, 190–204
    in Weekend Jump Start, 184
Food allergies, 46–47, 48–50, 127, 171, 286–287, 289
Food preferences, 42–43, 80–81
Foot care, 160–161, 274, 283, 297
Fortamet, 28–29
Free radicals, 18, 20, 51, 162
Freshness, of food, 83–88, 113
Fructose, 90, 168
Fruit
    benefits, 77–78, 90
    in controlling sweet cravings, 65–66
    dried, as snack, 114
    recipes
        Baked Apples, 262
        Chocolate-Covered Banana, 262
        Crustless Apple Pie, 263
        Fruit Smoothie, 264
        Marinated Peaches, 264
        Pineapple Mousse, 264
        Poached Pears, 265
        Red Currant Sauce, 267
    seasonal eating, 101
    shopping/storage tips, 255–261
    tropical, as pro-inflammatory, 92
Fungal infections, 274–275

G

Galvus, 30
Game meats, 103–104
Gardening, 152
Garlic, 131
Genetically modified organisms (GMOs), 60, 109
Genetics, 7, 21
Gestational diabetes, 4